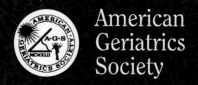 American Geriatrics Society

Geriatric Education FOR Emergency Medical Services

Resource Manual

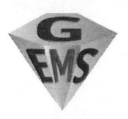

Lead Editor
Michael D. Panté, NREMT-P

Contributors
Russ Calhoun, BS, REMT-P
Bryan L. Fischberg, NREMT-P
Steven K Frye, BS, NREMT-P
Romeo Opichka, BBA, REMT-P
Michael D. Panté, NREMT-P
Stephen J. Rahm, NREMT-P
David L. Seabrook, MPA, EMT-P
Antonio Suarez, MSA, NREMT-P
Stephen H. Thomas, MD, MPH

JONES AND BARTLETT PUBLISHERS
Sudbury, Massachusetts
BOSTON   TORONTO   LONDON   SINGAPORE

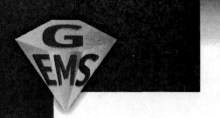

American Geriatrics Society
Executive Vice President: Linda Hiddemen Barondess
Associate Vice President, Professional Education and Special Projects: Nancy Lundebjerg, MPA
Senior Consultant, AGS Foundation for Health in Aging: Patricia Connelly
Manager, Professional Education and Special Projects: Linda Saunders
Manager, Professional Education and Special Projects: Dennise McAlpin

American Geriatrics Society
The Empire State Building
350 Fifth Avenue, Suite 801
New York, NY 10118
(212) 308-1414
www.americangeriatrics.org

Jones and Bartlett Publishers
World Headquarters
40 Tall Pine Drive
Sudbury, MA 01776
978-443-5000
info@jbpub.com
www.jbpub.com
www.GEMSsite.com

Jones and Bartlett Publishers Canada
6339 Ormindale Way
Mississauga, ON L5V 1J2
CANADA

Jones and Bartlett Publishers International
Barb House, Barb Mews
London W6 7PA
UK

Copyright © 2003 by American Geriatrics Society and Jones and Bartlett Publishers, Inc.

All rights reserved. No part of the material protected by this copyright may be reproduced or utilized in any form, electronic or mechanical, including photocopying, recording, or by any information storage and retrieval system, without written permission from the copyright owner.

The procedures and protocols in this book are based on the most current recommendations of responsible medical sources. The American Geriatrics Society and the publisher, however, make no guarantee as to, and assume no responsibility for, the correctness, sufficiency, or completeness of such information or recommendations. Other or additional safety measures may be required under particular circumstances.

This manual is intended as a guide to the appropriate procedures to be employed when rendering emergency care to the geriatric population. It is not intended as a statement of the standards of care required in any particular situation, because circumstances and the patient's physical condition can vary widely from one emergency to another. Nor is it intended that this textbook shall in any way advise emergency personnel concerning legal authority to perform activities or precedures discussed. Such local determination should be made only with the aid of legal counsel.

The GEMS course is a continuing education course; it is not a certification or licensure.
Notice: The patients described in the case studies throughout this text are fictitious.

Production Credits
Publisher: Kimberly Brophy
Associate Editor: Carol Brewer
Production Editor: Julie C. Bolduc
Senior Marketing Manager: Alisha Weisman
Manufacturing Buyer: Therese Bräuer
Cover Design: Shawn Girsberger and Kristin Ohlin
Printing and Binding: Odyssey Press
Cover Printing: Odyssey Press

ISBN-13: 978-0-7637-2207-8
ISBN-10: 0-7637-2207-7

Printed in the United States of America
11 10 09 08 07   10 9 8 7 6 5 4 3 2

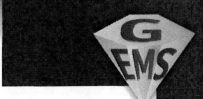

GEMS Steering Committee

David R. Snyder, MA, NREMT-P
Co-Chairperson, GEMS Steering Committee
Baltimore County Fire Department
Baltimore, Maryland

Colleen Christmas, MD
Co-Chairperson, GEMS Steering Committee
Representative from American Geriatrics Society
Johns Hopkins University
Baltimore, Maryland

Michael Armacost, MA, NREMT-P
Representative from National Association
   of State EMS Directors
Colorado Department of Health and Environment
Denver, Colorado

Roxy Barnes, RN
Representative from International Association
   of Fire Chiefs
Vancouver Fire Department
Vancouver, Washington

Heather Davis, MS, NREMT-P
Representative from National Association
   of EMS Educators
UCLA Center for Prehospital Care
Los Angeles, California

Barbara Dodge, BA, NREMT
Representative from National Council of State EMS
   Training Coordinators
Nebraska Department of Health and Human Services
Lincoln, Nebraska

John L. Esterhai, Jr, MD
Representative from American Academy
   of Orthopaedic Surgeons
University of Pennsylvania Medical Center
Philadelphia, Pennsylvania

Joann Freel, BS, CMP
Representative from National Association
   of EMS Educators
Carnegie, Pennsylvania

Tracy Haffer, RN
Representative from American Geriatrics
   Society
Johns Hopkins University
Baltimore, Maryland

Teresita M. Hogan, MD, FACEP
Representative from Society for Academic
   Emergency Medicine
Resurrection Medical Center
Chicago, Illinois

Richard C. Hunt, MD, FACEP
Representative from National Association
   of EMS Physicians
SUNY Upstate Medical University
Syracuse, New York

Michael O'Keefe, MS, NREMT-P
Representative from National Council
   of State EMS Training Coordinators
Vermont Department of Health
Burlington, Vermont

Michael D. Panté, NREMT-P
Member-at-Large
Robert Wood Johnson University Hospital
New Brunswick, New Jersey

Judith Ruple, PhD, RN, NREMT-P
Representative from National Association
   of EMS Educators
University of Toledo
Toledo, Ohio

LCDR Christopher Schmidt, NC, USN
Representative from Emergency Nurses
   Association
Naval Hospital
Jacksonville, Florida

David L. Seabrook, MPA, EMT-P
Representative from International Association
   of Fire Fighters
Vancouver Fire Department
Vancouver, Washington

Richard S. Slevinski, MD
Representative from American College
   of Emergency Physicians
Florida Emergency Medicine Foundation
Pace, Florida

Stephen H. Thomas, MD, MPH
Representative from National Association
   of EMS Physicians
Harvard Medical School and Massachusetts
   General Hospital
Cambridge, Massachusetts

Andy Trohanis, MA, EMT-B
Representative from National Council
   of State EMS Training Coordinators
Maryland Institute for Emergency Medical
   Services Systems
Baltimore, Maryland

Sue Fryer Ward, MSW, LCSW, BCD
Representative from National Association
   of State Units on Aging
Maryland Department of Aging
Baltimore, Maryland

Nathan Williams, EMT
Representative from National Association
   of Emergency Medical Technicians
Clinton, Mississippi

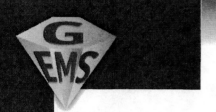

Contents

SECTION 1: ADMINISTRATION — 1

Who Should Take GEMS? — 3

Who Conducts GEMS Courses? — 3
- GEMS Course Coordinator — 3
- GEMS Faculty — 5

GEMS Course Schedules — 5
- Optional Lectures — 5
- BLS Course One-Day Schedule — 6
- BLS Course Modular Schedule (2 Sessions) — 7
- ALS Course One and One-Half Day Schedule — 8
- ALS Course Modular Schedule (3 Sessions) — 9

GEMS Course Preparation — 10
- Course Planning Checklist — 10
- Course Budget — 10
- Room Requirements — 11
- Course Equipment — 11
- Ordering Materials — 11
- Continuing Education Units — 13

Administering the GEMS Written Exam — 13
- Obtaining the Written Exam — 13
- Written Exam Security — 13
- Written Pre-Test — 13
- Written Post-Test — 13
- How to Administer the Written Post-Test — 13
- Scoring the Written Post-Test — 13
- Remediation — 13
- GEMS Course Completion Card — 14

GEMS Course Paperwork — 14
- Course Roster — 14
- Participant Evaluation Form — 14
- Faculty Evaluation Form — 14
- Course Coordinator Application — 14

GEMS Course Coordinator Orientation Session — 14
- Course Coordinator Prerequisites/Qualifications — 14
- Taking the Course Coordinator Orientation Session — 15
- Requirements for Conducting the Course Coordinator Orientation Session — 15
- Responsibilities Associated with the Course Coordinator Orientation Session — 15
- Course Coordinator Orientation Session Objectives — 15
- Course Coordinator Orientation Outline — 16

SECTION 2: LECTURES — 17

Lecture Overview — 18

Course Lectures — 20
- Aging — 20
- Changes with Age — 27
- Communicating with Older People and Their Caregivers — 36
- ALS: Assessment of the Older Patient — 44
- BLS: Assessment of the Older Patient and Pharmacology — 55
- End-of-Life Care Issues — 64
- Trauma, Musculoskeletal Disorders, and Falls — 70
- Neurological Emergencies and Altered Mental Status — 80
- Respiratory and Cardiovascular Emergencies — 91
- Elder Abuse and Neglect — 102
- ALS: Pharmacology and Medication Toxicity Emergencies — 110
- ALS: Psychiatric Emergencies — 120

BLS and ALS Optional Course Lectures — 128
- Other Medical Emergencies — 128
- Improving Quality of Life — 141

SECTION 3: SCENARIOS — 147

Scenarios Overview — 148

BLS Scenarios — 149
- Communication Challenges — 149
- Do Not Resuscitate Orders — 152
- Stroke — 154
- Medication Interactions — 157
- Elder Abuse and Neglect — 160
- Delirium vs. Dementia — 163

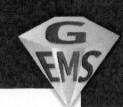

ALS Scenarios　166
 Communication Challenges　166
 Do Not Resuscitate Orders　170
 Stroke　172
 Medication Interactions　175
 Elder Abuse and Neglect　179
 Delirium vs. Dementia　182

SECTION 4: SKILL STATIONS　185

Skill Station Overview　186

BLS and ALS Skill Stations　188
 Conducting a Patient Assessment
  Interview　188
 Immobilization　209

Optional ALS Skill Station　224
 Intravenous Therapy　224

SECTION 5: APPENDIX　231

GEMS BLS Course Fact Sheet　232

GEMS ALS Course Fact Sheet　233

Course Notification Form　234

Course Coordinator Application　235

Course Coordinator Orientation
Session Confirmation Letter　237

Faculty Confirmation Letter　238

Participant Confirmation Letter　239

GEMS Faculty Evaluation Form　241

GEMS Participant Evaluation Form　243

GEMS Course Roster　245

Administration

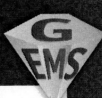

Section 1

Contents

- **Who Should Take GEMS?** 3
- **Who Conducts GEMS Courses?** 3
  - GEMS Course Coordinator 3
    - Prerequisites/Qualifications 3
    - The Course Coordinator Orientation Session 3
    - Maintaining Status as a Course Coordinator 4
    - Responsibilities 4
  - GEMS Faculty 5
    - Prerequisites/Qualifications 5
    - Responsibilities 5
    - Faculty-to-Participant Ratio 5
    - Preparation 5
- **GEMS Course Schedules** 5
  - Optional Lectures/Skills 5
  - BLS Course One-Day Schedule 6
  - BLS Course Modular Schedule (2 Sessions) 7
  - ALS Course One and One-Half Day Schedule 8
  - ALS Course Modular Schedule (3 Sessions) 9
- **GEMS Course Preparation** 10
  - Course Planning Checklist 10
  - Course Budget 10
  - Room Requirements 11
  - Course Equipment 11
  - Ordering Materials 12
  - Continuing Education Units 13
- **Administering the GEMS Written Exam** 13
  - Obtaining the Written Exam 13

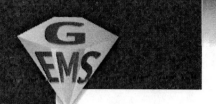

Section 1: Administration

- Written Exam Security 13
- Written Pre-Test 13
- Written Post-Test 13
- How to Administer the Written Post-Test 13
- Scoring the Written Post-Test 13
- Remediation 13
- GEMS Course Completion Card 14
- **GEMS Course Paperwork** **14**
  - Course Roster 14
  - Participant Evaluation Form 14
  - Faculty Evaluation Form 14
  - Course Coordinator Application 14
- **GEMS Course Coordinator Orientation Session** **14**
  - Course Coordinator Prerequisites/Qualifications 14
  - Taking the Course Coordinator Orientation Session 15
  - Requirements for Conducting the Course Coordinator Orientation Session 15
  - Responsibilities Associated with the Course Coordinator Orientation Session 15
  - Course Coordinator Orientation Session Objectives 15
  - Course Coordinator Orientation Outline 16

Section 1: Administration

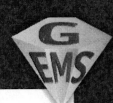

Administration

Who Should Take GEMS?

The primary audience for the GEMS course should be comprised of First Responders, EMTs, Paramedics, and other emergency care providers. In addition, health care professionals responsible for emergency care of older people will benefit from the course. GEMS is designed to address the special needs of the older population, including the geriatric objectives identified in the EMT-Basic, Intermediate, and Paramedic National Highway Traffic Safety Administration (NHTSA) National Standard Curricula.

GEMS offers a one-day basic life support (BLS) course and a one and one-half day advanced life support (ALS) course. The BLS course is designed for First Responders and EMT-Basics; the ALS course is designed for EMT-Intermediates and EMT-Paramedics. The Course Coordinator determines which course (BLS or ALS) is most appropriate for an individual.

Who Conducts GEMS Courses?

The GEMS course requires:
- GEMS Course Coordinator
- GEMS Faculty

NOTE: Follow your state or local protocols regarding medical oversight and/or direction.

GEMS Course Coordinator

Prerequisites/Qualifications
To be a Course Coordinator, an individual must meet the following prerequisites/qualifications:
- Be a physician (MD or DO), registered nurse, nurse practitioner, advanced practice nurse, physician assistant, paramedic, or EMT, with a background in EMS. (He or she must be at least a paramedic to coordinate a GEMS ALS course.)
- Successfully complete the GEMS provider course at the same or higher level for which the individual seeks to conduct courses.
- Submit the Course Coordinator application for approval to the Course Coordinator conducting the Course Coordinator Orientation Session or submit the application online at www.GEMSsite.com before completing the Online Course Coordinator Orientation Session.
- Have documented experience in conducting other nationally recognized standardized courses for prehospital personnel. The person also should have knowledge, experience, and expertise in the conduct of other adult education programs.
- Demonstrate an understanding and a working knowledge of the most recent GEMS course materials and policies.
- Complete any required updates on the GEMS course materials.

The Course Coordinator Orientation Session
Individuals who meet the prerequisites/qualifications to become a Course Coordinator will be eligible to attend a GEMS Course Coordinator Orientation Session or complete the Online Course Coordinator Orientation Session at www.GEMSsite.com. Additional information about these two options can be found in the section titled "GEMS Course Coordinator Orientation Session" on page 14.

Based on the individual's qualifications and which GEMS course he or she has completed, the individual will become a GEMS BLS and/or ALS Course Coordinator. The BLS Course Coordinator can conduct GEMS BLS courses and can lead orientation sessions for future BLS Course Coordinators. The ALS Course Coordinator can teach both BLS and ALS courses as well as the Course Coordinator Orientation Session for individuals seeking to become either BLS or ALS Course Coordinators.

The following chart outlines what GEMS BLS and ALS Course Cordinators are qualified to teach.

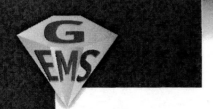

Section 1: Administration

Status	Qualified to Teach
BLS Course Coordinator	• GEMS BLS Course • Course Coordinator Orientation Session for BLS Course Coordinators
ALS Course Coordinator	• GEMS BLS Course • GEMS ALS Course • Course Coordinator Orientation Session for Course Coordinators

Maintaining Status as a Course Coordinator

An individual's Course Coordinator status is valid for two years. To renew this status, the individual must participate in at least two GEMS courses within the two-year period. This involvement can be either as a Course Coordinator or as Faculty at a registered course.

Responsibilities

The Course Coordinator is responsible for the quality of the GEMS course. Responsibilities include:

- Educational Quality—The Course Coordinator is responsible for the educational quality of the GEMS course and must ensure that the content is presented in its entirety. The Course Coordinator must provide oversight to assure that the course content and instructional program complies with the standards and guidelines set forth in the GEMS course curriculum.
- Course Supervision—The Course Coordinator must attend the entire course. He or she should supervise the registration process; observe lectures, scenarios, and skill stations; and be prepared to intervene if necessary (this may involve teaching a segment of the course or redirecting a scenario or skill station).
- Course Integrity—The quality of the GEMS course relies heavily on the Course Coordinator. He or she should maintain the integrity of the course and ensure that all minimum course requirements are met. The Course Coordinator must provide oversight to assure the quality of the educational experience and of the Faculty.
- Faculty Selection—The Course Coordinator is responsible for recruiting, preparing, and supervising the Faculty for the course being conducted. The Course Coordinator must provide oversight to assure the Faculty possesses the appropriate skills and knowledge required for presenting specific lectures. Additional information about Faculty prerequisites/qualifications and responsibilities is provided in the section titled "GEMS Faculty" on page 5.
- Coordinate Logistics—The Course Coordinator is responsible for all logistical issues, such as teaching materials, equipment, room reservations, registration, catering, and promotion. In some cases these responsibilities can be delegated. The section titled "GEMS Course Preparation" on page 10 provides more information on logistics.
- Budget Management—The Course Coordinator manages the course budget. The section titled "Course Budget" on page 10 provides more information on the GEMS course budget.
- Course Evaluations—The GEMS Steering Committee would like to continually improve the GEMS course; therefore, feedback from the course participants and Faculty is very important. The Course Coordinator should ensure all participants and Faculty members complete a course evaluation form. (The forms can be found in the Appendix.) Course Coordinators are required to submit the evaluation forms from the first course they coordinate and are encouraged to submit forms for every course they coordinate thereafter. Completed forms should be sent to the American Geriatrics Society (AGS) at the following address:

GEMS American Geriatrics Society
The Empire State Building
350 Fifth Avenue, Suite 801
New York, NY 10118
212-308-1414

- Course Roster Submission—At the completion of each GEMS course, the Course Coordinator needs to complete and send the course roster to the AGS. The section titled "Course Rosters" found on page 14 contains more information about course rosters.

Section 1: Administration

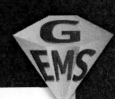

- Ensuring Safety—The Course Coordinator must ensure that universal safety precautions are followed.

GEMS Faculty

The Course Coordinator is responsible for selecting the Faculty for the course.

Prerequisites/Qualifications

To be considered for a position on the GEMS Faculty, an individual must meet the following requirements:
- Be a health care professional or allied health professional.
- Have teaching experience and knowledge of the scope and practice of prehospital medical services.
- Successfully complete the GEMS provider course at the level for which he or she wishes to teach.

Responsibilities

The GEMS Faculty have many important responsibilities that ensure a quality GEMS course. Faculty should possess the knowledge and skills necessary to teach the course, and shall:
- Facilitate Learning—Faculty should teach the assigned material in an engaging manner that facilitates the learning process of the participants in the course.
- Work with Course Coordinator and Other Faculty—Typically, a GEMS course involves one Course Coordinator and several Faculty members. It is essential that all the leaders work together to conduct a successful course, in a consistent manner.
- Be Familiar with Assigned Material—In order to be effective teachers, the Faculty must familiarize themselves with the course objectives and assigned material prior to the course.
- Read All Assigned Material—Faculty members will receive a copy of the GEMS Resource Manual and the GEMS Textbook prior to the course. They must read the sections pertaining to their teaching assignments and be prepared to present the material.

Faculty-to-Participant Ratio

In a GEMS course, the Faculty-to-participant ratio is 1:6; therefore, the number of Faculty needed depends upon the number of participants enrolled in the course. For example, if a course has 24 participants, a minimum of 4 Faculty members are needed.

Preparation

The Course Coordinator is required to meet with all Faculty prior to the start of the course in order to address:
- Course schedule
- Questions about course content
- Management of scenarios and skill stations
- Any unusual situations or potential irregularities and local protocol issues

GEMS Course Schedules

The content in the GEMS courses allow for a few scheduling options. The BLS course can be completed in a single day or divided into multiple modules. The ALS course can be completed in a day and a half or divided into multiple modules. The following charts suggest schedules for the various options. Please note that these sample schedules include minimum course content and minimum times. Depending upon time, interest, and target group, the course can be lengthened to include optional lectures/skills and to allow more time for participant practice or discussion.

Optional Lectures/Skills

The following optional lectures/skills can be added to a GEMS course. The optional IV therapy skill can be added for any provider level that allows this skill. The Course Coordinator should be certain to add time to the schedule for the additional lectures.

BLS Optional Lectures
- Psychiatric Emergencies
- Other Medical Emergencies
- Improving Quality of Life

ALS Optional Lectures
- Other Medical Emergencies
- Improving Quality of Life

Optional Skill
- Intravenous Therapy

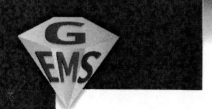

Section 1: Administration

BLS Course One-Day Schedule

Lecture	Aging	15 minutes
Video—Segment 1	Aging	10 minutes
Lecture	Changes with Age	30 minutes
Video—Segment 2	Communication and Assessment	10 minutes
Lecture	Communicating with Older People and Their Caregivers	30 minutes
Break		10 minutes
Lecture	Assessment of the Older Patient and Pharmacology	30 minutes

Concurrent Sessions (Scenarios and Skill Stations)

Scenarios	Communication Challenges	45 minutes
Skill Stations	Conducting a Patient Assessment Interview	(45 minutes)
Lunch		30 minutes
Lecture	End-of-Life Care Issues	15 minutes
Lecture	Trauma, Musculoskeletal Disorders, and Falls	30 minutes
Video—Segment 3	Immobilization	10 minutes
Lecture	Neurological Emergencies and Altered Mental Status	30 minutes
Break		10 minutes

Concurrent Sessions (Scenarios and Skill Stations)

Scenarios	Do Not Resuscitate Orders Stroke	30 minutes
Skill Stations	Immobilization	(30 minutes)
Lecture	Respiratory and Cardiovascular Emergencies	40 minutes
Lecture	Elder Abuse and Neglect	20 minutes
Scenarios	Medications Interactions Dementia vs. Delirium Elder Abuse and Neglect	40 minutes
Break		10 minutes
GEMS Written Exam		20 minutes

Total Time: 9 hours
Content Time: 8 hours (does not include breaks or lunch)

Section 1: Administration

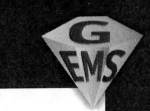

BLS Course Modular Schedule (2 Sessions)

Session 1

Lecture	Aging	15 minutes
Video—Segment 1	Aging	10 minutes
Lecture	Changes with Age	30 minutes
Video—Segment 2	Communication and Assessment	10 minutes
Lecture	Communicating with Older People and Their Caregivers	30 minutes
Break		10 minutes
Lecture	Assessment of the Older Patient and Pharmacology	30 minutes
Lecture	End-of-Life Care Issues	15 minutes

Concurrent Sessions (Scenarios and Skill Stations)

Scenarios	Communication Challenges	45 minutes
Skill Stations	Conducting a Patient Assessment Interview	(45 minutes)

Total Time Session 1: 4 hours
Content Time Session 1: 3 hours and 50 minutes (does not include breaks)

Session 2

Lecture	Trauma, Musculoskeletal Disorders, and Falls	30 minutes
Video—Segment 3	Immobilization	10 minutes
Lecture	Neurological Emergencies and Altered Mental Status	30 minutes
Break		10 minutes

Concurrent Sessions (Scenarios and Skill Stations)

Scenarios	Do Not Resuscitate Orders Stroke	30 minutes
Skill Stations	Immobilization	(30 minutes)
Lecture	Respiratory and Cardiovascular Emergencies	40 minutes
Lecture	Elder Abuse and Neglect	20 minutes
Scenarios	Medications Interactions Dementia vs. Delirium Elder Abuse and Neglect	40 minutes
Break		10 minutes
GEMS Written Exam		20 minutes

Session 2 Total Time: 4 hours and 30 minutes
Session 2 Content Time: 4 hours and 10 minutes (does not include breaks)

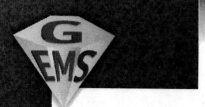

Section 1: Administration

ALS Course One and One-Half Day Schedule

Day 1

Lecture	Aging	15 minutes
Video—Segment 1	Aging	10 minutes
Lecture	Changes with Age	30 minutes
Video—Segment 2	Communication and Assessment	10 minutes
Lecture	Communicating with Older People and Their Caregivers	30 minutes
Break		10 minutes
Lecture	Assessment of the Older Patient	30 minutes

Concurrent Sessions (Scenarios and Skill Stations)

Scenarios	Communication Challenges	45 minutes
Skill Stations	Conducting a Patient Assessment Interview	(45 minutes)
Lunch		30 minutes
Lecture	End-of-Life Care Issues	15 minutes
Lecture	Trauma, Musculoskeletal Disorders, and Falls	30 minutes
Video—Segment 3	Immobilization	10 minutes
Lecture	Neurological Emergencies and Altered Mental Status	30 minutes
Break		10 minutes
Lecture	Respiratory and Cardiovascular Emergencies	40 minutes

Concurrent Sessions (Scenarios and Skill Stations)

Scenarios	Do Not Resuscitate Orders Stroke	30 minutes
Skill Stations	Immobilization	(30 minutes)

Total Time Day 1: 7 hours and 30 minutes
Content Time Day 1: 6 hours and 40 minutes (does not include breaks or lunch)

Day 2

Lecture	Elder Abuse and Neglect	20 minutes
Lecture	Pharmacology and Medication Toxicity Emergencies	45 minutes
Lecture	Psychiatric Emergencies	30 minutes
Break		10 minutes
Scenarios	Medication Interactions Dementia vs. Delirium Elder Abuse and Neglect	45 minutes
Video—Segment 4	Intravenous Therapy	10 minutes
GEMS Written Exam		20 minutes

Total Time Day 2: 3 hours
Content Time Day 2: 2 hours and 50 minutes (does not include breaks)

Total Time: 10 hours and 30 minutes
Total Content Time: 9 hours and 30 minutes (does not include breaks or lunch)

Section 1: Administration

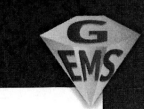

ALS Course Modular Schedule (3 Sessions)

Session 1

Lecture	Aging	15 minutes
Video—Segment 1	Aging	10 minutes
Lecture	Changes with Age	30 minutes
Video—Segment 2	Communication and Assessment	10 minutes
Lecture	Communicating with Older People and Their Caregivers	30 minutes
Break		10 minutes
Lecture	Assessment of the Older Patient	30 minutes

Concurrent Sessions (Scenarios and Skill Stations)

Scenarios	Communication Challenges	45 minutes
Skill Stations	Conducting a Patient Assessment Interview	(45 minutes)

Total Time Session 1: 3 hours and 45 minutes
Content Time Session 1: 3 hours and 35 minutes (does not include breaks)

Session 2

Lecture	End-of-Life Care Issues	15 minutes
Lecture	Trauma, Musculoskeletal Disorders, and Falls	30 minutes
Video—Segment 3	Immobilization	10 minutes
Lecture	Neurological Emergencies and Altered Mental Status	30 minutes
Break		10 minutes
Lecture	Respiratory and Cardiovascular Emergencies	40 minutes

Concurrent Sessions (Scenarios and Skill Stations)

Scenarios	Do Not Resuscitate Orders Stroke	30 minutes
Skill Stations	Immobilization	(30 minutes)

Total Time Session 2: 3 hours and 5 minutes
Content Time Session 2: 2 hours and 55 minutes (does not include breaks)

Session 3

Lecture	Elder Abuse and Neglect	20 minutes
Lecture	Pharmacology and Medication Toxicity Emergencies	45 minutes
Lecture	Psychiatric Emergencies	30 minutes
Break		10 minutes
Scenarios	Medication Interactions Dementia vs. Delirium Elder Abuse and Neglect	45 minutes
Video—Segment 4	Intravenous Therapy	10 minutes
GEMS Written Exam		20 minutes

Total Time Session 3: 3 hours
Content Time Session 3: 2 hours and 50 minutes (does not include breaks)

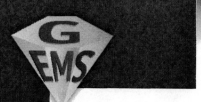

Section 1: Administration

GEMS Course Preparation

Advance preparation is a key factor to a successful GEMS course. It is recommended that Course Coordinators begin planning several months prior to the start date. The following checklist provides the information necessary for advance planning.

Course Planning Checklist

Prior to the course:
- Select which course to teach (ALS or BLS)
- Select course dates
- Reserve a location for the course
- Identify appropriate people to serve as Faculty (page 5)
- Develop course budget and set the registration fee (page 10)
- Mail Faculty Confirmation Letters (Appendix)
- Establish registration procedures
- Post the upcoming course on www.GEMSsite.com
- Develop a plan for promoting the course
- Order textbooks and other GEMS materials from Jones and Bartlett Publishers (1-800-832-0034)
- Make arrangements for course supplies and equipment (page 11)
- Reserve audiovisual equipment (page 11)
- Send the first mailing to prospective participants, using the GEMS course promotional piece available on www.GEMSsite.com
- Select the caterer and menus for lunch and breaks
- Schedule a meeting with Faculty
- Process registration
- Mail packages to course participants with confirmation letter, information about course location and parking facilities, as well as course materials, including the GEMS textbook (page 12). This should be done at least 2 weeks prior to the start of the course.

No later than one-day prior to the course:
- Set-up the registration area
- Set-up the rooms for skill stations and scenarios
- Hold Faculty meeting
- Photocopy GEMS Written Exam
- Confirm order with caterers

During the course:
- Check rooms and equipment prior to and immediately after each session
- Place course signs in appropriate locations
- Have staff available to answer questions and provide directions
- Facilitate course participant and Faculty registration
- Distribute evaluation forms to participants and Faculty (Appendix)
- Monitor course to maintain schedule and flow
- Monitor lectures, scenarios, and skill stations
- Check set-up for lunch and breaks
- Grade GEMS Written Exams
- Collect participant and Faculty evaluation forms

After the course:
- Submit the course roster and evaluation forms to the AGS (page 4)
- Submit Course Coordinator applications to the AGS if a Course Coordinator Orientation Session was conducted (page 15)
- Send appropriate paperwork to continuing education provider for approval
- Send thank you letters to Faculty and support staff
- Send Faculty an honorarium (optional)
- Return equipment
- Pay invoices

Course Budget

The cost of conducting a GEMS course varies depending on institutional/organizational support and the availability of facilities and equipment. To help defray costs, the GEMS Course Coordinator establishes a registration fee. In addition, the Course Coordinator may want to investigate sources of outside funding.

The following outline lists items the Course Coordinator needs to consider when planning a GEMS course budget.

Facility Expenses
- Rental fee for lecture hall and break-out rooms
- Catering charges for lunches and breaks*

*NOTE: The GEMS course does not mandate a requirement for supplying lunches and breaks.

Section 1: Administration

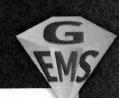

Equipment Purchase and Rental
- Equipment rental and disposable supplies for skill stations
- Audiovisual equipment

Faculty Expenses
- Faculty transportation, lodging, meals, and in some cases honorarium
- Continuing education credit application fees

Course Supplies
- GEMS Textbook for each participant and Faculty member
- GEMS Resource Manual for each Faculty member
- GEMS ToolKit CD-ROM or Slide Set
- GEMS Video
- GEMS Skill Station Notecards
- Name badges
- Registration supplies
- Photocopies of the GEMS Written Exam
- Photocopies of the GEMS Evaluations

Promotion
- Brochure development, design, printing, and mailing
- Advertisements
- Posters

Postage
- Participant and Faculty confirmation packages

Room Requirements

One large room is necessary for the lectures. Each participant needs a place to sit and, ideally, tables or desks would be available. The lecture room also must have the necessary audiovisual equipment, including a slide projector and a screen or computer with CD-ROM drive, an LCD projector, and a screen, and a VCR and television monitor.

Several break-out rooms are also necessary. The Faculty-to-participant ratio of 1:6 determines how many rooms are needed. The break-out rooms should be free from distractions to ensure that appropriate discussion and interaction can occur.

Course Equipment

The following outline lists the supplies and equipment needed for the GEMS BLS and ALS courses. At the beginning of each Skill Station (GEMS course Skill Stations can be found in the section titled "Skill Stations" on page 185), there is a list of the equipment needed for that particular station.

GEMS BLS or ALS Course Audiovisual Equipment
- Computer with CD-ROM drive
- LCD projector
- Screen for projecting slides

Or
- Slide projector
- Slide carousel
- Screen for projecting slides

- Television monitor
- VCR

Supplies
- GEMS Textbooks (one per participant and Faculty)
- GEMS Resource Manual (one per Faculty)
- GEMS ToolKit CD-ROM or Slide Set
- GEMS Video
- GEMS Skill Station Notecards
- GEMS BLS or ALS Written Exam (one per participant)
- GEMS Evaluations
- Name tags (one per participant and Faculty)
- Parking passes (if necessary)
- Signs
- Paper
- Pens

Skill Station 1—Conducting a Patient Assessment Interview
- Exam gloves (large, medium, and small) (latex-free if possible)
- Oxygen tank and oxygen administration supplies
- First aid kit including blood pressure cuff, stethoscope
- Medication bottles with simulated labels (hydrochlorthiazide, nitroglycerin, furosemide, and potassium)
- Ziploc bags
- Mouth guards or large gumballs
- Several pairs of earplugs
- Patient simulation materials:
  - Sunglasses with tape on lenses (can be plastic, nonprescription)
  - Yellow-tinted (or other color) sunglasses

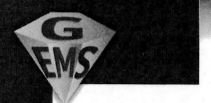

Section 1: Administration

Or
- Geriatric simulation kit
- Tattered clothes/robes
- Winter coat
- Stones/pebbles
- Gauze and tape
- RMA form (to practice signing with impaired mobility)
- Small pill-sized candies (such as Tic-Tacs)
- Photocopies of page from business section of phone book
- Dishwashing gloves
- Observer Handouts (photocopy from Skill Station section):
  - Conducting a Patient Assessment Interview—Situation 1:
    – Observing Students (page 193)
  - Conducting a Patient Assessment Interview—Situation 2:
    – Observing Students (page 199)
  - Conducting a Patient Assessment Interview—Situation 3:
    – Observing Students (page 205)

Skill Station 2—Immobilization
- Exam gloves (large, medium, and small) (latex-free if possible)
- Oxygen tank and oxygen administration supplies
- First aid kit including blood pressure cuff, stethoscope
- Long board
- Scoop stretcher
- Cervical collars (various sizes)
- Head blocks/head bed immobilization device
- Straps/tape
- Padding to fill void spaces (blankets, pillows, or commercial device)
- Medication bottles with simulated labels (Lasix, Lanoxin)
- Stuffed animal cats/dogs
- Fake eggs and milk
- Mouth guards or large gumballs
- Several pairs of earplugs

- Patient simulation materials:
  - Sunglasses with tape on lenses (can be plastic, nonprescription)
  - Yellow-tinted (or other color) sunglasses

Or
- Geriatric simulation kit
- Towels or small pillows
- T-shirt
- Observer Handouts (photocopy from Skill Station section)
  - Immobilization—Situation 1:
    – Observing students (page 213)
  - Immobilization—Situation 2:
    – Observing students (page 219)

Optional Equipment
- Wheelchair
- Cane
- Immobilization vacuum mattress
- Commercial inflatable backboard pillow
- Rhythm simulator
- Cardiac monitor/ECG

Ordering Materials

The following GEMS materials are available through Jones and Bartlett Publishers:
- GEMS Textbook (ISBN: 0-7637-2086-0)
- Resource Manual (ISBN: 0-7637-2270-7)
- ToolKit CD-ROM (ISBN: 0-7637-2271-5)
- Slide Set (ISBN: 0-7637-2272-3)
- Video (ISBN: 0-7637-2273-1)
- Teaching Package with ToolKit CD-ROM (ISBN: 0-7637-2269-3)
- Teaching Package with Slide Set (ISBN: 0-7637-2268-5)

To order materials, contact Jones and Bartlett Publishers:
Phone: 800-832-0034
Fax: 978-443-8000
Online: www.GEMSsite.com

Section 1: Administration

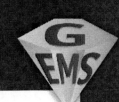

Continuing Education Units

Course Coordinators need to work with the appropriate agency in their region or state to secure continuing education units for the GEMS participants. The AGS is not able to award continuing education units. If Course Coordinators are not certain about how to secure continuing education units, they should contact the state EMS office.

Administering the GEMS Written Exam

The GEMS written exam is an important part of determining whether participants have mastered the material and course objectives presented in the GEMS course. The following sections provide the details needed for administering the GEMS written exam.

Obtaining the Written Exam

GEMS Course Coordinators receive the GEMS written exam packets when they successfully complete the GEMS Course Coordinator Orientation Session. BLS Course Coordinators should receive only BLS materials. The GEMS written exam packet contains the following:

- BLS Pre-Test
- BLS Pre-Test Answer Key
- BLS Post-Test Version 1
- BLS Post-Test Version 1 Answer Key
- BLS Post-Test Version 2
- BLS Post-Test Version 2 Answer Key
- ALS Pre-Test
- ALS Pre-Test Answer Key
- ALS Post-Test Version 1
- ALS Post-Test Version 1 Answer Key
- ALS Post-Test Version 2
- ALS Post-Test Version 2 Answer Key

Written Exam Security

It is the responsibility of the GEMS Course Coordinator to ensure the security of the GEMS written exam. Participants in a GEMS course should not be permitted to leave the course with a copy of a GEMS written exam or answer key. Likewise, while Faculty can assist with the administration of the GEMS written exam, they should not be given their own copy or be permitted to leave the course with a copy of the GEMS written exam or answer key.

Written Pre-Test

It is optional to administer the pre-tests contained in the exam packets for the BLS and ALS GEMS courses. Pre-tests are often useful in determining the knowledge level of the participants. If the Course Coordinator elects to administer the pre-tests, appropriate time must be added to the schedule.

Written Post-Test

Each participant wishing to receive a GEMS Course Completion Card must successfully complete the GEMS written exam for the appropriate level (BLS or ALS).

How to Administer the Written Post-Test

The GEMS written exam is administered at the end of a GEMS course. Participants who attended all components of the course are eligible to take the exam. It is a closed-book exam and is corrected by the Course Coordinator or Faculty member. Prior to the course, the Course Coordinator is responsible for photocopying the correct post-test and answer key.

Scoring the Written Post-Test

The GEMS written exam packet includes an easy-to-use answer key. The following table provides the passing scores.

Exam	Number of Questions	Minimum Score to Pass
BLS Post-Test	20	16 (80%)
ALS Post-Test	25	20 (80%)

Remediation

Some participants will not pass the GEMS written exam on the first attempt. In these cases, the Course Coordinator works with them to develop a remediation plan. Together, they should review the questions that the participant missed and discuss the material.

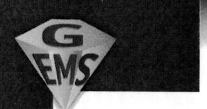

Section 1: Administration

The participant may take the GEMS written exam a second time, preferably on another day, as it is unlikely that the participant will improve his or her knowledge enough to pass on the same day. However, the Course Coordinator should use discretion and allow retesting on the same day if circumstances warrant. For the second attempt, the alternate version of the GEMS written exam should be given. If the participant does not pass again, he or she must retake the course to receive a GEMS Course Completion Card.

GEMS Course Completion Card

The GEMS course is a continuing education course designed to provide education. It does not certify or license participants.

Participants who successfully complete the BLS or ALS GEMS course qualify to receive an American Geriatrics Society GEMS Course Completion Card, which is valid for two years. To receive this card, the participant must:
- Participate in the entire course
- Pass the GEMS written exam

GEMS Course Paperwork

The Course Coordinator must complete the following forms and submit them to the AGS.

Course Roster

It is important for the AGS to keep a record of participants in the GEMS courses. At the conclusion of a course, the Course Coordinator must complete the GEMS course roster. Course Coordinators can submit a roster via the GEMS website at www.GEMSsite.com for no charge. There is a $20.00 processing fee per roster for Course Coordinators who wish to submit a course roster to the AGS via fax or mail. After a completed course roster is received by the AGS, course completion cards will be sent to the Course Coordinator.

Participant Evaluation Form

The Course Coordinator is responsible for ensuring that each participant completes a GEMS participant evaluation form. The form with instructions for completion can be found on page 243.

Course Coordinators must submit participant evaluation forms to the AGS the first time they conduct a course, and they are encouraged to submit forms for every course thereafter. The Course Coordinator should make copies of the participant evaluation forms in order to remember suggestions for future courses.

Faculty Evaluation Form

The Course Coordinator is also responsible for ensuring that Faculty members complete a GEMS faculty evaluation form. Again, Course Coordinators are required to submit faculty evaluation forms to the AGS the first time they conduct a course, and they are encouraged to submit the forms for every course they conduct thereafter. The faculty evaluation form with instructions for completion can be found on page 241.

The Course Coordinator should make copies of the faculty evaluation forms before they are submitted to the AGS in order to improve their future courses.

Course Coordinator Application

Any Course Coordinator is qualified to prepare other individuals to become Course Coordinators. The candidates must complete the Course Coordinator application found on page 235. Applications should be submitted to the AGS via the GEMS web site at www.GEMSsite.com for no charge, or to the AGS via fax or mail for a $20.00 processing fee.

GEMS Course Coordinator Orientation Session

The GEMS Course Coordinator Orientation Session is designed to prepare GEMS providers to serve as GEMS Course Coordinators.

Course Coordinator Prerequisites/Qualifications

A person must meet the following requirements to qualify to attend a GEMS Course Coordinator Orientation Session.
- Be a physician (MD or DO), registered nurse, nurse practitioner, advanced practice nurse, physician assistant, paramedic, or EMT, with a background in EMS. (He or she must be at least a paramedic to coordinate a GEMS ALS course.)

Section 1: Administration

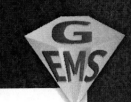

- Successfully complete the GEMS provider course at the same or higher level for which the individual seeks to conduct courses.
- Submit the Course Coordinator application for approval to the Course Coordinator conducting the Course Coordinator Orientation Session or submit the application online at www.GEMSsite.com before completing the Online Course Coordinator Orientation Session.
- Have demonstrated experience in conducting other nationally recognized standardized courses for pre-hospital personnel. The person also should have knowledge, experience, and expertise in the conduct of other adult education programs.
- Demonstrate an understanding and a working knowledge of the most recent GEMS course materials and policies.

Taking the Course Coordinator Orientation Session

GEMS providers enrolled in the Course Coordinator Orientation Session will need the following materials:
- GEMS Textbook
- Resource Manual

Requirements for Conducting the Course Coordinator Orientation Session

- Have conducted at least one GEMS course, serving as the Course Coordinator.

Responsibilities Associated with the Course Coordinator Orientation Session

The responsibilities of the GEMS Course Coordinator conducting the Course Coordinator Orientation Session include:
- Verify that each GEMS provider participating in the Course Coordinator Orientation Session meets the requirements to become a GEMS Course Coordinator.
- Send a Course Coordinator Orientation Session confirmation letter to the GEMS providers who will be participating in the Course Coordinator Orientation Session. A sample Course Coordinator Orientation Session confirmation letter can be found on page 237. This letter should provide information on how the participant can obtain a copy of the Resource Manual or a copy of the Resource Manual can accompany the letter.
- Prepare for teaching the Course Coordinator Orientation Session by arranging for classroom space and audiovisual needs.
- Ensure that participants have read the Resource Manual prior to the Course Coordinator Orientation Session.
- Ensure that participants have completed the Course Coordinator application prior to the Course Coordinator Orientation Session.
- Teach Course Coordinator Orientation Session, following the orientation session schedule. To teach the orientation session, Course Coordinators will need:
  - ToolKit CD-ROM or print-out from www.GEMSsite.com
  - Course Roster
- Upon completion of the Course Coordinator Orientation Session, submit orientation session roster and course coordinator applications via the GEMS web site at www.GEMSsite.com, fax, or mail to the AGS for each applicant. The course roster with instructions for completion can be found on page 245. The Course Coordinator application with instructions for completion can be found on page 235.

Course Coordinator Orientation Session Objectives

At the conclusion of the Course Coordinator Orientation Session, participants will be able to:
- List the types of students who should take the GEMS course.
- Specify who can teach the GEMS course.
- Describe the requirements for becoming a GEMS Course Coordinator.
- Define the qualities that Faculty of a GEMS course must possess.
- Organize the steps necessary to conduct a GEMS course.
- Successfully conduct a GEMS course.
- Define the successful completion for a student completing the GEMS course.
- Explain the post-course paperwork required to complete the GEMS course.
- Identify the requirements to continue serving as a GEMS Course Coordinator.
- Summarize the steps necessary to complete a GEMS Course Coordinator Orientation Session.

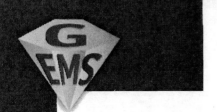

Section 1: Administration

Course Coordinator Orientation Outline

The following outline provides an overview and timetable for the Course Coordinator Orientation. The Course Coordinator conducting the orientation needs to verify that the participants meet the criteria to become a GEMS Course Coordinator *before* the orientation begins.

Time	Content
5 minutes	Welcome and Introductions
3 minutes	Overview of Orientation Objectives
12 minutes	The GEMS Course and Personnel
6 minutes	Preparation and Materials
3 minutes	GEMS Course Schedules
6 minutes	Components of the GEMS Course
3 minutes	Course Completion
21 minutes	GEMS Website
6 minutes	GEMS Course Forms
2 minutes	Continuing Education
9 minutes	Course Coordinator Orientation
2 minutes	Exams
2 minutes	Course Coordinator Status

Total Time: 80 minutes

For more information on becoming a GEMS Course Coordinator, visit the GEMS website at www.GEMSsite.com.

Lectures

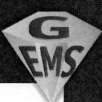

Section 2

Russ Calhoun, BS, REMT-P
Bryan L. Fischberg, NREMT-P
Steven K. Frye, BS, NREMT-P
Romeo Opichka, BBA, REMT-P
Michael D. Panté, NREMT-P
Stephen J. Rahm, NREMT-P

Contents

- **Lecture Overview** 18
- **Course Lectures** 20
    - Aging 20
    - Changes with Age 27
    - Communicating with Older People and Their Caregivers 36
    - ALS: Assessment of the Older Patient 44
    - BLS: Assessment of the Older Patient and Pharmacology 55
    - End-of-Life Care Issues 64
    - Trauma, Musculoskeletal Disorders, and Falls 70
    - Neurological Emergencies and Altered Mental Status 80
    - Respiratory and Cardiovascular Emergencies 91
    - Elder Abuse and Neglect 102
    - ALS: Pharmacology and Medication Toxicity Emergencies 110
    - ALS: Psychiatric Emergencies 120
- **BLS and ALS Optional Course Lectures** 128
    - Other Medical Emergencies 128
    - Improving Quality of Life 141

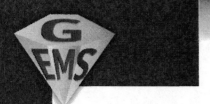

Section 2: Lectures

Lecture Overview

Lecture Outline Format and Features

The lectures included in the GEMS course schedule are:
- Aging
- Changes with Age
- Communicating with Older People and Their Caregivers
- Assessment of the Older Patient and Pharmacology (BLS)
- Assessment of the Older Patient (ALS)
- End-of-Life Care Issues
- Trauma, Musculoskeletal Disorders, and Falls
- Neurological Emergencies and Altered Mental Status
- Respiratory and Cardiovascular Emergencies
- Elder Abuse and Neglect
- Pharmacology and Medication Toxicity Emergencies (ALS)
- Psychiatric Emergencies (ALS)

In this section, the actual slide content is presented on the left, with the accompanying lecture script for the Faculty on the right. Note that the lecture script provides additional information that the Faculty may wish to use to understand the concepts better or to enhance their presentation. The Faculty presenting lectures in the course should also read the accompanying chapter(s) from the GEMS textbook, as this resource provides more in-depth information about each subject than is provided in this section.

The lecture script is presented in bulleted statements. There is one slide every 1 to 2 minutes, and the presenting Faculty should pace themselves to ensure that each lecture finishes on time.

Special instructions to the Faculty are presented in ***bold italics*** in the additional information. Using these suggestions will result in a more effective and interesting lecture, and are only a starting point. Faculty may bring additional personal experience to enhance the lectures further.

The lectures in the GEMS course include case studies. Generally, content is presented and then followed by case studies in which students apply the knowledge, serving to reinforce learning and improve retention. Some case studies are presented gradually throughout the lecture, when appropriate. It is more difficult to implement a case-based lecture, but many times students find such lectures more interesting and informative because information is presented in the context for which they practice.

Teaching tips specific to each lecture are provided at the beginning of each outline for the Faculty's convenience, and to facilitate team teaching and student interaction.

Finally, be sure to follow along with the course schedule you have chosen so that the video segments are shown at the appropriate times in between lectures and skill station/scenario concurrent sessions.

ALS Content

The GEMS course is available as a BLS or ALS course. Some lectures are used in both the BLS and ALS course, while others are customized specifically for the BLS or ALS course. For example, there are different assessment lectures for the BLS and ALS courses.

Section 2: Lectures

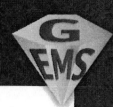

ALS content is marked on slides with the same ALS icon found in the GEMS textbook. Note that this content is presented on both the BLS and ALS slides. While BLS providers are not trained to perform ALS skills, the ALS information has been provided for their edification in this continuing education course.

On the ToolKit CD-ROM, BLS and ALS lectures are organized into separate folders for your convenience. If you are using the 35mm Slide Set in lieu of the PowerPoint presentations included on the ToolKit CD-ROM, note that ALS slide presentations are provided on red slide mounts. When presenting a BLS course, remove the red slides. When presenting an ALS course, use the red slides.

Optional Lectures

There are two optional lectures provided in this section:
- Other Medical Emergencies
- Improving Quality of Life

These lectures cover Chapters 12 and 15 from the GEMS textbook. These lectures can be presented to BLS or ALS audiences if you wish to run a longer, more comprehensive course.

Note that the Psychiatric Emergencies lecture included in the ALS course schedule can be presented as an optional lecture in the BLS course as well.

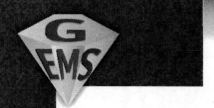

Section 2: Lectures

Aging

Teaching Tips

The Aging lecture serves to start the course. It is important to capture the students' attention immediately, as the first lecture sets the tone for the entire course. It is also important to create opportunities for interaction in this lecture so students feel engaged and understand that they can ask questions and actively participate throughout the rest of the course.

A good way to encourage student interaction is to ask specific questions at various points during the lecture. Sometimes these questions can be open-ended, giving students the chance to brainstorm. At other times, the questions can be more specific to the content. For example, to open this lecture, you could ask, "What comes to mind when you think of older people?" Allow a brief session for responses. Then move on to introduce the course. Later in the lecture, you could ask students questions regarding specific content, such as, "Why is it important to use a respectful tone with older patients?" or "How could a rude or condescending tone from the EMS provider affect an emergency call involving an older patient? In the case studies, you may ask students, "What should you do for this patient?"

The lecture can also be customized with your personal experience. At various points in the lecture, adding tips from your field experience or stories about an emergency call with an older patient can engage students and drive the point home. You may also ask students about their experiences with older people—since this is continuing education, most providers attending the course will already have some experience with older people and may be able to share their own tips regarding interaction and care.

Immediately following this lecture, show video Segment 1: Aging.

Lecture Outline: Aging

Slide Text	Additional Information
Slide #1 **Aging**	This lecture covers topics found in Chapter 1: Aging. *Before beginning this lecture, catch the students' interest. Tell a story about a personal experience you have had with an older patient. Ask students if their grandparents or other older relatives have ever needed to call EMS. Ask students why younger people sometimes have negative attitudes towards older people.* *Tell students that EMS is the first and sometimes only help available to older patients. Older people have special needs that need to be considered during assessment, communication, and treatment.*

Section 2: Lectures

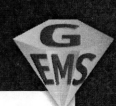

Slide Text	Additional Information
Slide #2 **Objectives** • Describe the concept of the GEMS diamond. • Discuss the social aspects of aging. • Describe negative stereotyping of older people. • Describe the living arrangements of older people.	*Read objectives.*
Slide #3 **The GEMS Diamond** • Remember the following when caring for older people: – Geriatric patients – Environmental assessment – Medical assessment – Social assessment	The GEMS diamond was created to help you remember what is different about the older patient. Keep this in mind whenever you go on a call involving an older patient. Table 1-5 lists the components of the GEMS diamond in greater detail. "G" stands for geriatric. The first thing you should think of when you go on a call involving an older patient is that older patients are different and may present atypically. Remember the changes that occur with age (taught in the Changes with Age lecture), and remember that an older person is as human as a child or younger adult. Treat them with respect and dignity. "E" stands for environmental assessment. The environment may contain clues to the cause of the emergency. Is the home well kept and secure? Are there hazardous conditions (poor lighting, throw rugs, poor wiring, broken windows)? Is the home too hot or too cold (taking into account an older person's sensitivity to temperature)? *Ask students if they have encountered a hazardous environment in an older person's home.* "M" stands for medical assessment. Older patients tend to have a variety of medical problems, and may be on numerous prescription and OTC medications. Obtain a thorough medical history. "S" stands for social assessment. Older people may have less of a social network, due to the death of a

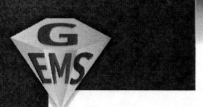

Section 2: Lectures

Slide Text	Additional Information
	spouse or moving away of family members, or friends. This can lead to depression. The older person may need additional help with activities of daily living (ADLs) but may not have anyone to help. Find out if the patient has sufficient social support to care for both physical and emotional needs. Be alert for signs of elder abuse and neglect. ***Ask students if they have encountered socially isolated patients.***
Slide #4 **Aging Statistics** • 13% of people in the US are over age 65. • "Baby Boomers" will increase this number. • Expect to see an increase in emergency calls involving older patients.	The number of older patients is on the rise. People are living to older ages and remaining more active throughout their lifespan. In the year 2000, nearly 13% of the population was over age 65. This number is expected to increase, peaking around the year 2030. "Baby Boomers," those born following the second world war, make up a large portion of the population. These "Boomers" will be entering the older population, forcing the numbers of people 65 and above to swell. With this increased population, EMS can surely expect to see an increase in need for care. Currently, approximately 41% of the population over age 65 require ambulance transport. The five states with the highest percentage of population over age 65 (See Fig. 1-3): Florida 18.3% Penn. 15.4% Iowa 15.3% RI & WV 15.0%
Slide #5 **Case Study** • Dispatched to a residence for an 84-year-old woman who has fallen • Patient, Mrs. Reed, cannot get up.	Your service is dispatched for an 84-year-old woman named Mrs. Reed who fell. The call comes in as "fallen and can't get up". The address is in a well-established neighborhood with an aging population. Your service is dispatched to this neighborhood often as many are retired and do not have easy access to emergency health care other than through EMS.

Section 2: Lectures

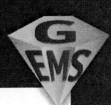

Slide Text	Additional Information
	Ask class: "Right off the bat, what do you think of when you receive this kind of call?" *(Elicit answers.)* Throughout your assessment consider the GEMS diamond. Geriatric concerns for this patient should include why the patient fell. Is there a medical cause to the problem? Is there trauma from the fall? Could this be a case of neglect? Consider the whole picture during the rest of your exam.
Slide #6 **Case Study (continued)** • En route your partner says, "Oh no, not another 'I can't get up' call!" *Is this attitude healthy?*	*Read slide.* *(Elicit answers from the class.)* This attitude is negative.
Slide #7 **Case Study (continued)** • Mrs. Reed is on the kitchen floor. • She is alert but weak. • S: States she fell last night • Has pain in left hip • Vital signs are normal.	You arrive to find Mrs. Reed lying on the kitchen floor. Her son states he found her on the floor, unable to move. She answers questions appropriately, but makes no effort to move or sit on her own. She states that she tripped last night at dinner time and was unable to get to the phone. (Consider "S" in the GEMS diamond.) She complains of pain in the left hip and says that she felt a pop when she fell. The left leg is rotated externally. Vital signs are a blood pressure of 124/84 mm Hg, a pulse of 88 beats/min, respirations of 18 breaths/min, skin is warm and dry, pulse Ox is 97% on room air, and the ECG is normal sinus rhythm. Her blood sugar is 110 mg/dL and her neurological exam is normal with decreased movement of left leg due to pain.
Slide #8 **Ageism** • Stereotyping and discrimination of older people • Categorizing people as senile, eccentric, or stubborn	Ageism is stereotyping and discriminating against people because of their age. Older people are commonly categorized as senile, comical, eccentric, stubborn or unable to learn new things. These classifications are often accentuated by how our society looks at getting older. Being forgetful, walking with

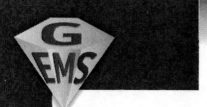

Section 2: Lectures

Slide Text	Additional Information
• "Geezer," "Lizard," and "GOMER" perpetuate ageism • Use of "honey" or "dear" is a milder form	a cane or walker, having difficulty with one's hearing or eyesight are individual problems and not issues related to the older generation.
Slide #9 **Living Arrangements** • Most live at home. • Women are more likely to live alone. • Less than 5% are institutionalized.	The living arrangements of older persons will vary. Most (67%) live in a family setting. Men over age 65 often live with a spouse. However, women are more likely to be widows and live alone. Only 4.3% of the population over age 65 lives in an institutional setting. This percentage increases with age.

Slide #10
Case Study (continued)
• You conduct a GEMS exam:
  – **E:** Small amounts of food, home is warm and clean
  – **M:** No significant medical history, no medications
  – **S:** Son reports that mother lives alone, no regular contact with friends
	Remembering "E" in the GEMS diamond, you notice only small amounts of food around the kitchen. You see no pots or pans despite the fact that the patient fell just after dinner last night. You inquire about eating habits and the patient tells you that she usually has a banana and toast for breakfast, a bowl of bran cereal for lunch, and vegetables and a potato for dinner.
	
	When questioned about her medical history ("M" in the GEMS diamond), the patient reveals that she does not go to a doctor regularly because she has always been very healthy.
	
	Your social exam ("S" in the GEMS diamond) shows an older woman who has lived alone since her husband died three years earlier. She has no regular friends, and her son is her only family. He comes over once a week to help with chores and shopping.

Section 2: Lectures

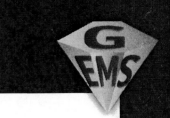

Slide Text	Additional Information
Slide #11 **Access to Essential Services**<ul><li>Transportation</li><li>Meal preparation</li><li>Health care</li><li>Social activities</li></ul>	Older people often have difficulty accessing services essential to everyday activities. Transportation to and from shopping, doctor's office visits, the pharmacy, or the laundromat may be limited by the cost of operating a vehicle or losing one's license due to disabilities. Rising costs of electric, gas, or other utilities can limit heat, the use of a stove for cooking, or hot water for bathing. Access to health care can be limited by transportation, but also by cost for someone on a fixed income. Getting out for social interaction can be limited by cost, transportation, or the ability to meet with others in the same situation.
Slide #12 **Case Study Conclusion**<ul><li>Mrs. Reed is transported to ED.</li><li>Report to Social Services for potential follow up.</li></ul>	You give Mrs. Reed information on local transportation services funded by the community. Mrs. Reed is transported to the ED for evaluation of a hip fracture. You leave a verbal report with the ED staff regarding the patient living alone and possibly needing help. Social services follows up with you during the next week to advise you that they were able to arrange a home health aid several times a week, that "Meals on Wheels" will be delivering hot meals 3 times a week, and the county transportation service will be arranging for the patient's transportation needs for shopping and other trips.
Slide #13 **Summary**<ul><li>Number of people over age 65 is rising</li><li>Older people have many social and environmental concerns.</li></ul>	Care of the older patient requires the EMS provider to look not only at immediate illness or injury, but also at the overall health of the patient. Being an advocate for older patients requires EMS providers to evaluate social and environmental factors in their patients' lives. Active participation against ageism within EMS and the community must be attained.

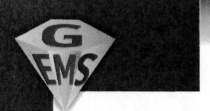

Section 2: Lectures

Slide Text	Additional Information
• We must understand and accept aging. • Family remains the most common residence for the older population.	By understanding the aging process and accepting the consequences of aging, we can better help our patients.

Section 2: Lectures

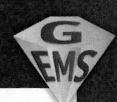

Changes with Age

Teaching Tips

This lecture provides a foundation for understanding what makes older people different physically. This information will help students understand why older people require different medical care. It will help students understand why their interaction with older people needs to be modified in order to be effective. It will also teach how the physical changes a person experiences as he or she ages can create different or increased risks for illness or injury.

As you proceed through this lecture, remember to incorporate the GEMS diamond into your presentation whenever possible. This concept will help unify the course, but will not be as effective if it is not used in all lectures. In each lecture, the GEMS diamond is incorporated on slides where it is applicable, and also in all case studies. When you see the GEMS diamond, be sure to discuss how it applies at this point in the lecture.

Much of the content in this lecture in particular may be new to BLS providers. When presenting this lecture to a BLS audience, allow more time for students to ask questions. Be sure to present the general concepts in a clear and understandable way, with language that is appropriate for the BLS provider. Instead of expounding on higher-level topics, use extra time for clarifying material and answering questions. As a general rule throughout the course, always be sure to adjust your presentation to your audience.

Lecture Outline: Changes with Age

Slide Text	Additional Information
Slide #1 **Changes with Age**	This lecture covers topics found in Chapter 2: Normal Changes with Age.
Slide #2 **Objectives** • List the major diseases and disorders common to older people. • Identify the general decline in organ systems in the older person.	*Read objectives.*
Slide #3 **Objectives (continued)** • Explain the changes brought about from aging in physical structure, body composition, and organ function. • Define normal psychological changes affecting older people.	*Read objectives.*

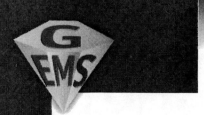

Section 2: Lectures

Slide Text	Additional Information
Slide #4 **Leading Causes of Death in Older People** • Disease of the heart • Cancer • CVA/Stroke • COPD • Pneumonia	The leading causes of death in older people give us a clue to the conditions that we will see as EMS providers caring for the older population. Institutions such as the American Diabetes Association list heart disease as the leading cause of diabetic deaths.
Slide #5 **Case Study** • Dispatched for 79-year-old man with difficulty breathing • Says he always gets winded easily and cannot catch his breath today • E: Environment is clean and warm.	You are dispatched to the home of a 79-year-old male, Mr. Brophy, complaining of difficulty breathing. Mr. Brophy appears in moderate distress with retractions and nasal flaring, and he gets 4 to 5 words out before becoming winded. He states that he gets winded easily, but today he just can't catch his breath. He is sitting upright in a chair, has taken two puffs on his inhaler, and increased his oxygen from 2 L/min to 3 L/min. The environment is clean and warm.
Slide #6 **Case Study (continued)** • History of AMI, CHF, COPD, hypertension, diabetes • Pulse = 112 beats/min • Respirations = 28 breaths/min • Blood pressure = 160/96 mm Hg • **ALS**: ECG = A-fib • **ALS**: Pulse Ox = 92% on oxygen	Mr. Brophy states a history of an AMI three years earlier, CHF, emphysema from a long history of heavy smoking, high blood pressure that is controlled by medication, and adult onset diabetes. Vital signs are a pulse of 112 mm Hg, respirations of 28 breaths/min and labored, and a blood pressure of 160/96 mm Hg. **ALS:** The ECG shows atrial fibrillation, and pulse Ox is 92% on 3 L/min with his home O_2.
Slide #7 **Case Study (continued)** *What factors influence how well Mr. Brophy can compensate for his illness?* G: *How will aging affect these factors?*	*What factors influence how well Mr. Brophy can compensate for his illness?* *(Elicit answers.)* Factors affecting compensatory mechanisms include: ability to ventilate, ability to respire, ability to circulate blood, and ability of the nervous system to sense the changes required to stimulate a ventilation. *How will aging affect these factors?* Each of these systems will change with normal aging (consider "G" in the GEMS diamond).

Section 2: Lectures

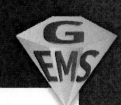

Slide Text	Additional Information
Slide #8 **The Aging Body: Integumentary System** • Wrinkles • Thinner skin • Decreased fat • Gray hair	The normal changes with age will be discussed system-by-system, starting with the outside (the skin). The skin is the first thing that we see when we meet an older person. Wrinkles appear as the skin becomes thinner, drier, and less elastic. Elastin and collagen decrease and fibrin builds up, making skin less pliable. The subcutaneous fat layer thins out over time, resulting in little cushion to absorb bumps and bruises. Finally, hair becomes thinner and gray. Gray hair is produced by the lack of melanin in the hair follicle. Decreases in melanin produce a hair without pigment, seen as gray.
Slide #9 **The Aging Body: Respiratory System** • Changes in airway • Decreasing muscles of ventilation • Increased residual volume • Decreased sensitivity of chemoreceptors	Changes in the respiratory system start in the physical structure of the airway. Aging dentition or dental replacements, such as bridges or dentures, can make airway obstruction more prominent. The cilia that line the airway decrease in number, causing less cough reflex when foreign bodies enter the lower airway. The smooth muscle that lines the airway weakens with age. This can cause the airway to swell or collapse with the positive and negative pressures of ventilation. Muscles of the chest wall also weaken, leaving less ability to compensate for increased workload. **ALS:** The alveoli become larger, but decrease in total number. The alveoli that are left are often scarred by the effects of smoking or pollutants. This leaves less surface area for gas exchange. Residual volume increases with age due to less pliable lung tissue, chest wall, and alveoli. With less movement of the lungs, air is left at the end of expiration and stagnant air remains in the lungs.

Section 2: Lectures

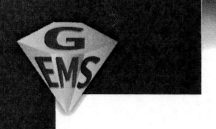

Slide Text	Additional Information
	This can cause the body to become slightly hypercarbic and a related acidosis can develop.
	The chemoreceptors, which monitor the blood for carbon dioxide levels, become slower with age. This slowing affects the speed of impulses to the diaphragm that triggers each breath. This slowing can be seen in a lowered normal pulse Ox reading of 93% to 95% on room air.
Slide #10 **The Aging Body: Cardiovascular System** • Development of atherosclerosis • Decreasing cardiac output • Development of arrhythmias • Changes in blood pressure	The whole cardiovascular system is affected by the development of atherosclerosis. With the thickening of the vessel walls, there is lessened ability to compensate by constricting or dilating the vessels during trauma or hypotensive events. The heart will need to push blood flow through these stiffened vessels, leading to hypertension and hypertrophy over time.
	The heart muscle, like all of the other muscles, will begin to weaken with age. Cardiac output [CO = Stroke volume (SV) × Heart rate (HR)] decreases as a result of the stroke volume decreasing from weakening muscles. Rate-limiting medications or arrhythmias can also affect the cardiac output.
	The conductive system of the heart will see decreases of pacemaker cells. This is most prominent in the SA node where a decrease of 90% of the cells may be lost by age 75. The AV node cells will decrease as well, leaving the potential for arrhythmias including atrial fibrillation, AV nodal blocks, and junctional rhythms.
	Blood pressure becomes harder to regulate due to several factors. The baroreceptors, or pressure sensors, monitor the pressure in the body. These receptors, located in the aortic arch, become less sensitive with age, allowing greater swings in pressure to occur before sending a message to the brain to change the pressure. On top of that, the message

Section 2: Lectures

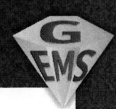

Slide Text	Additional Information
	is then sent through an aging nervous system. The effect is a slowed response to pressure changes. This is apparent in older patients who feel dizzy when they get up too quickly. Also, atherosclerosis affects the body's ability to change the peripheral vascular response needed to regulate pressure. Peripheral vascular resistance plays an important role in changing pressure. The older trauma patient with hypotension due to blood loss has little ability to compensate well with the decreased cardiac output of an aging heart and the decreased response of the vasculature. With medications, the patient's ability to compensate may be even further limited.
Slide #11 **The Aging Body: Nervous System** • Brain shrinkage • Slowing of peripheral nerves • Slowed reflexes • Decreasing pain sensation	The brain will shrink throughout life, as much as 20% by age 80. Space develops in the subdural area, forcing the bridging veins to stretch. Trauma to the head can cause bleeding into this space (subdural hematoma) that may go unnoticed when looking for signs of head injury because ICP will not rise until the space has been filled. This is often too late to be managed effectively. Also, neurons decrease, producing less transfer of information throughout the brain. This is not to say that the brain slows (because it doesn't), but that it has a hard time moving the information. The peripheral nervous system slows, causing changes in the sensory and motor routes. Decreased sensation and slowed reflexes are a contributing cause of trauma in older people. Decreasing pain sensation is one of the reasons that classical presentations to medical complaints are altered or absent. A common condition may be the older patient with cardiac pain complaining only of respiratory distress or a toothache.

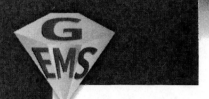

Section 2: Lectures

Slide Text	Additional Information
Slide #12 **Case Study (continued)** • G: Mr. Brophy appears to have a hard time hearing your questions. • Does not respond to all of your requests. *What are the sensory changes found in older patients?*	*Read slide.* *What are the sensory changes found in older patients?* **(Elicit answers.)**
Slide #13 **The Aging Body: Sensory Changes** • Vision distorts and eye movement slows. • Hearing loss is more common. • Taste decreases.	Eye movement and pupillary reaction slow with age. Peripheral fields narrow and a sensitivity to glare can develop. The opacity of the lens of the eye decreases and the lens thickens, making it harder to focus. Taking a history from an older patient is best done in front of them, at eye level. Hearing loss is about four times more common than loss of vision. Most older patients report loss of the higher frequencies. Taste sensation decreases, making food bland and unappetizing. This can contribute to malnutrition.
Slide #14 **Case Study (continued)** • S: Mr. Brophy reports feeling "down" lately. • S: Lives alone and has few friends still around *Is this patient at risk for depression?*	Mr. Brophy reports feeling "down" lately and not having much energy to get up and cook, clean, or go out. He lives alone since his wife passed away 2 years ago, and has outlived most of his friends. He has no other family in the area (consider "S" in the GEMS diamond). *Is this patient at risk for depression?* **(Elicit answers.)** Yes.
Slide #15 **The Aging Body: Psychological Changes** • Depression • Anxiety • Adjustment disorders	The stresses faced by older people, such as illness, physical limitations, and social loss can produce psychological changes. Though these changes are not normal, they can be seen more frequently in older people. Depression and anxiety disorders are often associated with medical conditions or medication usage. These often lead to adjustment disorders with demanding or controlling behavior on the part of the older adult.

Section 2: Lectures

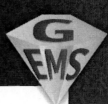

Slide Text	Additional Information
	Also, after retirement, people may experience a lost sense of identity and have trouble adjusting. Depression and suicide are a major concern in older patients. These patients tend to use more lethal means of suicide; use of firearms is the most common method.
Slide #16 **Case Study (continued)** **M:** When asked about medications, Mr. Brophy directs your attention to a shoebox. *How does the body react to medications with aging?*	When asked about his medications, Mr. Brophy points to a shoebox filled with medications (consider "M" in the GEMS diamond). *How does the body react to medications with aging?* **(Elicit answers.)**
Slide #17 **The Aging Body: Renal, Hepatic, and GI Systems** • Kidneys become smaller. • Hepatic blood flow decreases. • Production of enzymes declines. • Salivation decreases. • Gastric motility slows.	In the renal system, the kidneys become smaller (as much as 20%), lose nephrons, and function less. Aging kidneys also respond more slowly to increased demands put on the body. Many drugs are eliminated through the urine, including digoxin, lithium, and most antibiotics. The amount of blood that the liver can process decreases over time. Hepatic metabolism is affected by this decrease in flow and in the liver's diminished ability to produce and use metabolic enzymes. Medication levels are more likely to be harder to regulate with these changes. The gastrointestinal system ages from one end to the other. Salivation decreases, limiting the body's carbohydrate breakdown. Gastric motility slows, making constipation a likely issue in older patients. Blood flow through the mesentery arteries drops by as much as 50%, limiting the ability to extract the nutrition from the intestine. Finally, the anal sphincter loses elasticity, making fecal incontinence (and diapers) a greater possibility.

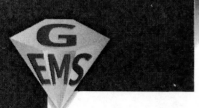

Section 2: Lectures

Slide Text	Additional Information
Slide #18 **The Aging Body: Musculoskeletal System** • Decreased muscle mass • Changes in posture • Arthritic changes • Decrease in bone mass	The musculoskeletal system sees tremendous changes during the later years. Muscle mass decreases over time and will be replaced by fat. The muscle fibers become smaller and fewer, and strength decreases. Decreases in muscle mass and atrophy of supporting structures produce postural changes. One of the most common is kyphosis, or hunchback. Shoulders move anteriorly and medially, the head and neck move anteriorly, and the upper thoracic spine becomes pronounced. Ligaments and cartilage lose elasticity and cartilage goes through degenerative changes contributing to arthritis. Bone loss or osteoporosis is seen in older patients of both sexes. However, it is seen more often in post-menopausal women. It can be the cause of hip fractures, vertebral body collapse, or other fractures.
Slide #19 **The Aging Body: Immune System** • Less effective immune response • Pneumonia and UTI are common. • Increase in abnormal immune system substances	Systemic and cellular immune responses become less effective. Pneumonia and urinary tract infections are common in bed bound patients. There are often abnormal immune system substances leading to increased incidence of infection in older people.
Slide #20 **Case Study Conclusion** • Mr. Brophy is treated for exacerbation of COPD. • Admitted to hospital, found to be on interacting medications • On discharge, Mr. Brophy was given follow-up visits with a home care service.	*Read slide.*

Section 2: Lectures

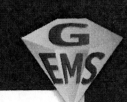

Slide Text	Additional Information
Slide #21 **Summary (1 of 2)** • Diseases common to the older population are familiar to EMS. • Organ systems decline in the aging body.	*Read slide.*

Slide #22
Summary (2 of 2)
• Aging body has:
  – Decrease in muscle and bone
  – Change in body structure
  – Less ability to compensate for stress
• Psychological changes:
  – Often caused by stress encountered in older population
	Read slide.

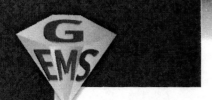

Section 2: Lectures

Communicating with Older People and Their Caregivers

Teaching Tips

Before starting this lecture, show video Segment 2: Communication and Assessment.

At this point in the course, the students will have been sitting for 50 minutes. Consider starting this lecture with a brief stretching session to get students invigorated and refocused.

This lecture is not clinical in nature but is absolutely critical in teaching students how to communicate with older people. Communication can be a major area of difficulty between EMS providers and older people. It can mean the difference between finding out what is really going on and providing appropriate treatment, or never realizing the underlying problem, such as depression, suicidal intent, social isolation, abuse, or neglect. The EMS provider may be the only person to whom the older person has access, and is therefore a critical link in the older person's health care.

In this lecture, it is a good idea to tie-in material from Lecture 2: Changes with Age. For example, you could state, "Recall that in the previous lecture, we learned about changes in vision and hearing that occur with age, as well as psychological changes. How might you need to adjust your communication skills to accommodate for these changes?"

This lecture is another great opportunity to get students involved. Ask plenty of questions. Find out what experiences (positive or negative) students have had communicating with older people. Discuss why younger people may feel negatively towards older people—it may be because of their own fears about growing old. Since this is a continuing education course, students will likely already have experiences, and perhaps even tips, that they can share with the class to enhance learning.

Lecture Outline: Communicating with Older People and Their Caregivers

Slide Text	Additional Information
Slide #1 Communicating with Older People and Their Caregivers	*At this point in the course, consider starting this lecture by asking students to stand up and stretch for a minute. This can help students refocus.* This lecture covers topics found in Chapter 3: Communicating with Older People and Their Caregivers.

Section 2: Lectures

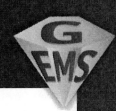

Slide Text	Additional Information
Slide #2 **Objectives** • Discuss principles and strategies for communicating effectively. • Recognize communication challenges with older patients. • Recognize the emotional need for independence in older people.	*Read objectives.*
Slide #3 **Objectives (continued)** • Describe common fears of older patients that interfere with effective communication. • Discuss recognizing and responding to caregiver stress.	*Read objectives.*
Slide #4 **Case Study 1** • Dispatched to "Unknown medical—older female patient" • 72-year-old Mrs. Weisman lying supine on living room floor • **E:** Room is dimly lit.	You are dispatched to the home of a 72-year-old woman, Mrs. Weisman, who is lying supine on the living room floor, in no apparent distress. The home is very neat and clean. The patient has lived here for 30 years, the first 25 with her husband and the last five by herself. You note that the room is dimly lit and remember the "E" in the GEMS diamond.
Slide #5 **Case Study 1 (continued)** • Family found patient after no phone call • Patient alert, oriented • Patient does not know why she is on floor. • Pulse = 88, Respirations = 18, BP = 126/84, pulse Ox = 96% • No trauma noted on exam. • Patient politely refuses your help.	Family came over to the check on patient after she did not answer the phone. They found the patient lying on the living room floor. She is alert and oriented but does not know why or how she ended up on the floor. Vital signs are a pulse of 88 beats/min, respirations of 18 breaths/min, a blood pressure of 126/84 mm Hg, and a pulse Ox of 96%. Your rapid trauma assessment reveals no trauma noted. The patient politely refuses your help and thanks you for coming.

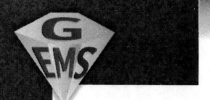

Section 2: Lectures

Slide Text	Additional Information
Slide #6 **Case Study 1 (continued)** • When you speak, the patient says, "What did you say?" • She is squinting her eyes. *How should you respond to older patients with diminished sight or hearing?*	When you speak with the patient, she turns her head and says, "What did you say?" As she looks toward you, she is squinting her eyes. *How should you respond to older patients with diminished sight or hearing?* **(Elicit answers.)**
Slide #7 **Communication Strategies** • Position yourself face to face. • Turn lights on. • Assist with glasses or hearing aids. • Use touch to calm and reassure. • Do not assume that blind means deaf. • Speak to good ear, raise volume, and lower pitch of speech.	Position yourself face to face at the patient's level. Turn on lights to help. Ask about eyeglasses and hearing aids. Assist the patient in putting them on. If the patient's vision is very poor, or if the patient is blind, stay close to the patient at all times, touch the patient as indicated to comfort and reassure, and never assume that a blind patient is also deaf or hard of hearing. Don't shout or yell! Speak louder and lower the pitch of your voice. Talk closely to the ear that can hear better. Try the reverse stethoscope technique if additional assistance is needed. Also, refer to Table 3-1 in text.
Slide #8 **Aphasia** • Inability to understand or produce speech • Can affect ability to read and write • Due to brain injury • Use focused, simple questions. • Give patient time to talk. • Use gestures and visual aids.	Aphasia is the inability to understand or produce speech. It is caused by brain injury. It is important to recognize aphasia when you encounter it in older patients. Refer to Tables 3-4 and 3-5. If you encounter a patient with aphasia, try the following: • Ask a family member or caregiver if the difficulty is with listening or talking, and modify your approach depending on the answer. • Talk to the patient as an adult, not a child. • Avoid open-ended questions; use focused questions. • Minimize background noise.

Section 2: Lectures

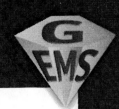

Slide Text	Additional Information
	• Get the patient's attention before communicating. • Encourage any kind of communication. • Keep your communication simple. • Give the patient time to talk. • Use gestures and visual aids when possible.
Slide #9 **Common Fears** *What are some common fears of older people that may affect how we communicate with them?*	*What are some common fears of older people that may affect how we communicate with them?* **(Elicit answers.)**
Slide #10 **Common Fears that Can Decrease Communication** • Loss of independence • Never leave hospital • Nursing home • Separation anxiety • Pet care and household security • Medical expenses	Older people feel comfortable and secure in their homes or "home-type" environment. They may stay longer than is safe for them, or avoid leaving, because they fear losing their independence, self-control, and their daily routine activities and schedule. They fear that they may worsen in the hospital, possibly die, become disabled or less functional, or be placed in a nursing home. Older people also fear being separated from their spouse, other family members, or friends. They become greatly concerned about their pets ("Who will feed and care for them while I'm gone?") and the security of their home (from burglary, or security of important records from "greedy/nosy" family members or relatives). Older people also worry about the additional medical bills and expenses.
Slide #11 **Case Study 1 Conclusion** • Address vision (eyeglasses). • Speak to "better" ear, lower pitch. • Recommend follow-up evaluations for eyes and ears. • Address her fear of losing independence.	You are able to locate the Mrs. Weisman's eyeglasses and assist her with placing them on her face. Her basic visual acuity is poor, even with the glasses. You determine that the Mrs. Weisman is deaf in one ear, has no hearing aid, and has never sought medical attention for it. You are able to speak

Section 2: Lectures

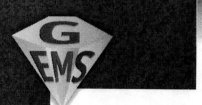

Slide Text	Additional Information
• Arrange for pets and home security. • Mrs. Weisman is transported to ED for further evaluation.	toward her "better" ear and lower the pitch of your voice. Though Mrs. Weisman is not significantly injured, her pronounced fear of losing her independence and control of her daily routine is preventing her from accepting your help. Talk with her about her fears. Her physician may be able to reevaluate her medications or hold a patient care conference with other physicians and family members to improve her care. Local programs may be able to assist her in remaining at home. After a somewhat lengthy discussion involving the patient, your medical director by cell phone, and her family, the patient agreed to your care and to transport to the emergency department. A trusted neighbor agrees to take care of her pets, and to secure the house and watch after it until she returns home.

Slide #12
Case Study 2
• Dispatched to agitated older male
• Stressed woman introduces husband:
  – **G:** Has a history of Alzheimer's, diabetes, hypertension
  – Appears frustrated, irritable, restless
	You arrive at your call location on a clear, pleasant weekday afternoon and are escorted into a clean, well-kept home by a neatly-dressed older woman who appears stressed, somewhat "frantic," as if she has been crying.
	
	She takes you to the living room, where she introduces you to her older husband, Mr. Chen, sitting on the sofa. She states that he has a history of recently worsening Alzheimer's disease, of diabetes and hypertension, and he takes several related medications (consider "G" in the GEMS diamond). He appears frustrated, irritable and restless, and he is mumbling in a disorganized manner.
	
	Communicating with Mr. Chen is difficult, but you and your partner are able to calm him down and complete a physical exam, revealing vital signs that are within normal limits.

Section 2: Lectures

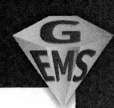

Slide Text	Additional Information
Slide #13 **Case Study 2 (continued)** • Vital signs are normal • No apparent injuries • Blood glucose: 112 mg/dL • **M:** Medications are given on prescribed schedule. • Mrs. Chen states, "I don't think I can continue to manage him without help!"	Per Mrs. Chen and your physical exam of Mr. Chen, there are no apparent injuries. Mr. Chen had earlier accidentally knocked over some potted plants on a patio table, and became very excited and agitated. When his hyperagitated state failed to resolve in its usual, relatively brief manner, Mrs. Chen called 9-1-1. Mr. Chen's blood glucose revealed 112 mg/dL. Mrs. Chen confirms that she administers his medication per the prescribed schedule. Remember the importance of medication adherence in older people, "M" in the GEMS diamond. As you are documenting your findings, Mrs. Chen drops her head down, covers her face with her hands and states "You probably need to check my blood pressure; I don't think I can continue to manage him without help!"
Slide #14 **Case Study 2 (continued)** *What are your concerns or findings thus far?* *What further questions would you ask in your assessment?*	*What are your concerns or findings thus far?* **(Elicit answers.)** Mr. Chen's dementia will likely complicate communication with him, making the assessment somewhat difficult. Also, if his agitation escalates, you may need to call for more assistance to safely manage Mr. Chen. *What further questions would you ask in your assessment?* **(Elicit answers.)** Has there been any injury to either party, given the initial call information? What happened? What is Mr. Chen's normal behavioral baseline?
Slide #15 **Recognizing Caregiver Stress or "Burnout"** • Physical effects on caregiver • Emotional effects on caregiver • Effects on "patient" and other family members	The caregiver may become physically exhausted or medically run down from ignoring his or her own medical and physical needs. The caregiver may also become emotionally "drained" or exhausted due to either the condition and demands of the patient, or due to failing to

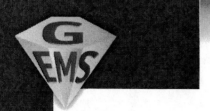

Section 2: Lectures

Slide Text	Additional Information
• Reducing caregiver stress • More than one patient?	find time to meet their own personal emotional needs. If the caregiver is not able to "keep up" with the demands of the patient, as well as their own needs, then the condition of the patient may suffer. Other family members, also dependent on the caregiver for attention and support, will find themselves "left out," and additional unexpected problems will arise within the family unit. Possibly, neglect and/or abuse of the patient or other family members may result. If caregiver stress seems apparent, briefly assess the caregiver's medical, psychological, and emotional states, in addition to assessing and managing the patient. If needed, based on your assessment, advise the caregiver of relevant options to improve their condition. Other family members, support groups or local agencies that assist seniors and their caregivers may be helpful resources. Consult your dispatcher or supervisor regarding a list of available support agencies and useful community support options. It might be best for the caregiver to ride to the receiving facility with the patient, so that appropriate support resources (social services and/or medical evaluation of the caregiver) may be identified and initiated immediately. Remember that some calls involving older people may involve more than one patient! Even if the situation does not seem like an emergency to you, the patient or caregiver felt it was enough of an emergency to call for help.

Section 2: Lectures

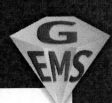

Slide Text	Additional Information
Slide #16 **Case Study 2 Conclusion** • Mr. Chen determined to be okay • Mrs. Chen assessed for caregiver stress • Mrs. Chen receives help from family • Doctor appointment for Mrs. Chen • Local "senior support" agency contacted with patient consent • Trusted neighbor offers to help • The Chens remain home.	You and your partner determine that Mr. Chen was not in need of medical attention at the moment, after he calmed down to his normal baseline state. You advise your supervisor and dispatch that you will have an extended scene time in order to evaluate Mrs. Chen, who appears overly stressed. Your assessment of Mrs. Chen, however, reveals a slightly elevated BP, a recent history of increasing insomnia, fatigue and weight loss, and poor eating habits. She also describes steadily increasing isolation and withdrawal from good friends and other family members. She denies that she is abusing alcohol or prescription medication. You are able to assist Mrs. Chen in obtaining [at least] a few days of assistance and support from a nearby family member, and, she is able to call and schedule an appointment with her family doctor for the day after tomorrow. Your supervisor assists you by contacting a local senior support agency, which calls Mrs. Chen while you are still "on scene." After consulting with your online medical control, you leave Mr. and Mrs. Chen at home, with a trusted neighborhood friend assisting them until their niece arrives later that evening. As you depart, you advise Mrs. Chen and the neighbor to call 9-1-1 again, if needed. In a few days, you call ahead to Mrs. Chen while on duty and drop by with your partner to visit with her and Mr. Chen, and to check on their progress.
Slide #18 **Summary** • Communication challenges • Principles of effective communication • Emotional need for independence • Common fears of older patients • Caregiver stress	*Review slide.*

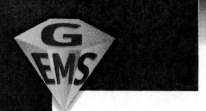

Section 2: Lectures

(ALS) Assessment of the Older Patient

Teaching Tips

This lecture is specifically designed for an ALS audience. It does not cover medication assessment or pharmacology, as the BLS assessment lecture does. Pharmacology is covered in its own separate lecture in the ALS GEMS course.

This lecture highlights the main points that are different in assessing an older patient. Be sure to emphasize that the assessment process does not change for an older patient. Students should still conduct the scene size-up, initial assessment, focused history and physical exam, detailed physical exam if applicable, and ongoing assessment.

This lecture also briefly discusses the top ten chief complaints of older patients, in order to familiarize students with the emergencies they will most likely encounter with this population.

Be sure to tie-in the material from Lecture 2: Changes with Age, as it relates to the material presented here. This can be done with statements such as, "Remember that in Lecture 2, we learned that older people are more sensitive to temperature due to thinning of the skin and loss of fat."

Lecture Outline: Assessment of the Older Patient

Slide Text	Additional Information
Slide #1 Assessment of the Older Patient	This lecture covers topics found in Chapter 5: Assessment of the Older Patient.
Slide #2 Objectives • Describe normal and abnormal assessment findings. • Recognize common emotional and psychological reactions. • Describe common complaints in the older patient.	*Read objectives.*
Slide #3 General Patient Assessment • E: Scene size-up includes environmental assessment: – General appearance, cleanliness – Temperature, food – S: Drugs, alcohol, signs of abuse	Patient assessment follows the same format taught in your initial training. However, there are several factors that differ in assessing the older patient. Scene size-up includes a thorough assessment of the environment. This is the "E" component of the GEMS diamond.

Section 2: Lectures

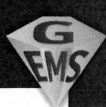

Slide Text

- Initial assessment looks for life threats:
  - Airway cannot be protected as well.
  - Breathing can be complicated by previous disease.
  - Circulatory system has slowed responses.

Additional Information

Look at the patient's general appearance. Can the patient dress, clean, and groom himself or herself without help? Does he or she have help if needed? This will begin to tell you how the patient manages their activities of daily living (ADLs). This is "S" in the GEMS diamond.

Pay attention to the temperature in the home. A cold home may indicate that the patient cannot afford to pay heating bills. Food is another indicator of how the patient manages financially. A lack of food will place the patient at risk for nutritional deficiencies.

Look around for signs of drugs, alcohol, or signs of abuse. Alcohol is a commonly abused substance for the older population. Signs of abuse may present as lack of care for the patient.

Initial assessment looks for life threats. These threats differ slightly in the older population. The airway is not protected as well as in younger people. Dentures, bridges, and other dental appliances can come loose and become an airway obstruction. The cilia that line the airway decrease in number, which allows easier aspiration of material.

Observing breathing can be complicated by previous disease. For example, a COPD patient would not be expected to have good chest rise with a barrel-shaped chest.

The circulatory system has slowed responses to stimuli. The older patient may have decreased pulses due to the changes in the vessels; the decreased pulse may not necessarily be due to the present illness.

Slide #4
Mental Status Assessment

- Confusion is not normal.
- Distinguish chronic changes from new ones.

During your assessment of the mental status, there are some things to remember.

Confusion is not normal. Changes in mentation require additional assessment.

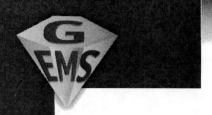

Section 2: Lectures

Slide Text	Additional Information
• Enlist help from family. • Establish a baseline mental status. • Don't be misled.	Determine chronic changes from new changes. This can often be done with one question: "What is different today?" Enlist the help of family or caregivers. These are the people that know the patient's norms and can help you to determine the changes. Establish a baseline mental status. Changes in mentation are dynamic. You will often be called during an evolving episode. Be able to relate what your baseline was. Don't be misled. A patient who is showing early signs of dementia may try to divert your attention from your exam of his or her orientation. When asked about the day, his or her reply may be "Why should I have to know that!" The question was not answered and the provider may feel reluctant to ask again. Persist in your questioning in a kind but firm manner—it is important to address the pride and fear of the patient so that you obtain the needed information.
Slide #5 **Assessment** • Prioritize patient status. • Detailed physical exam • Ongoing assessment is required.	Before moving on with your assessment, you need to determine your patient's priority for transport. Table 5-1 lists several reasons why your patient may need rapid transportation. The detailed physical exam should be completed according to your patient's status. Unstable patients should have an exam done en route to the hospital, while less urgent patients should be examined before transport to minimize distractions. During your exam, issues related to thermal regulation may be a problem. Older patients will often wear multiple layers of clothing and when removed or opened up, they may become cold. Take measures to keep the patient comfortable while performing your exam; for example, only expose what you need to expose in order to perform your exam. Ongoing assessment is more important with older patients compared to their younger counterparts.

Section 2: Lectures

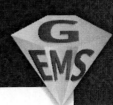

Slide Text	Additional Information
	Deterioration in the older patient's condition may be rapid. Vital signs should be taken every 15 minutes for a stable patient, while an unstable patient should have them taken every 5 minutes.
Slide #6 **Case Study 1** • Dispatched for an 82-year-old woman acting strangely; patient does not know why you are there. • Daughter states mother has Alzheimer's.	Your service is dispatched for a patient who is acting strangely. You begin to assess an 82-year-old woman, Mrs. Randish, who does not know why you are there. The daughter states that her mother has Alzheimer's disease and is acting strangely.
Slide #7 **Case Study 1 (continued)** • Daughter tells you that her mother is not listening today. • **G:** She tells you that her mother has had a cold. • **G:** Mrs. Randish is febrile, pale, and dry. *How would you approach the assessment of this patient?*	The daughter continues by telling you that her mother is not listening today. She has asked her to do several tasks this morning, but her mother has not done any of them. She tells you that her mother has had a cold for a couple of days. Mrs. Randish is febrile and her skin is pale and dry. Consider the "G" in the GEMS diamond, what might this presentation mean in an older patient? *How would you approach the assessment of this patient?* **(Elicit answers.)**
Slide #8 **Case Study 1 (continued)** • Pulse = 96 beats/min • Respirations = 24 breaths/min • BP = 110/70 mm Hg • Pulse Ox = 90% • Lungs have crackles in the lower left side. • Hands are cold.	Mrs. Randish's vital signs are a pulse of 96 beats/min, respirations of 24 breaths/min, a blood pressure of 110/70 mm Hg, and a pulse Ox of 90%. Lung sounds have crackles in the lower left lung. Her hands are cold.

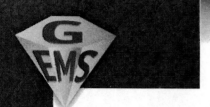

Section 2: Lectures

Slide Text	Additional Information
Slide #9 **Case Study 1 (continued)** • Signs include increasing agitation per daughter. • Allergic to sulfa • Medications include: Aricept, Paxil • Past history of Alzheimer's disease • Last meal was breakfast • Events are increasing agitation since this morning.	The case continues with a SAMPLE history. *(Read slide.)*
Slide #10 **Case Study 1 (continued)** • Mrs. Randish is becoming irritated with your questions. • Daughter is able to calm patient down. • Patient agrees to treatment and transport.	Mrs. Randish becomes irritated with your history taking and begins to talk loudly and act physically uptight. The daughter steps in and is able to calm the patient down. The patient agrees to be transported to the hospital.
Slide #11 **Case Study 1 Conclusion** • Mrs. Randish is given oxygen to bring saturation into mid 90's. • **ALS:** IV, cardiac monitor, 200 mL fluid bolus • Transported to the hospital, diagnosed with pneumonia. • Treated and released after 1 week	This case concludes with Mrs. Randish receiving oxygen, and IV fluids if an ALS unit is available. She was transported to the hospital and treated for pneumonia. The original complaint of "acting strangely" was not necessarily the patient's primary problem.
Slide #12 **Case Study 2** • Dispatched to a park to evaluate a 79-year-old man, Mr. Peterson, for difficulty breathing • He was taking his daily walk, became short of breath	Your service is dispatched for a 79-year-old man, Mr. Peterson, with difficulty breathing. He states he was taking his daily walk around the park when he became short of breath. He is speaking in short sentences, using accessory muscles, and sweating profusely.

Section 2: Lectures

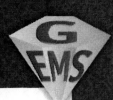

Slide Text	Additional Information
Slide #13 **Case Study 2 (continued)** *Is there a respiratory problem?* *Does the problem always match the complaint?*	*Is this a respiratory call?* **(Elicit answers.)** The answer is maybe, but not always. It could be cardiac, medication reaction/interaction, or fatigue. *Does the problem always match the complaint?* **(Elicit answers.)** Use the question to introduce the topic of complaint-based assessment.
Slide #14 **Assessing the Chief Complaint** • Determining the chief complaint can be hard. • Start with what is bothering the patient most. • Chief complaints may not be the life threat. • Communication is a big component.	The chief complaint may be difficult to determine due to multiple disease processes or multiple complaints. It is often easier to ask the patient what is bothering him or her today. The chief complaint is not always the life threat. For example pain from swollen feet may be fluid back up from CHF. Taking time to allow good communication between the caregiver and the patient is a major part of assessment. Complaints may need to be examined one-by-one in order to determine the patient's condition.
Slide #15 **Chief Complaint: Shortness of Breath** • Frequently life threatening • Often respiratory or cardiac in origin • Can occur for other reasons such as pain, bleeding, medications • Are there associated signs and symptoms? • Does patient have a history of respiratory complaints?	The next ten slides look at the top ten complaints made by older people seeking medical attention. These topics are listed by frequency, from more common to less. The complaint of shortness of breath can often be misleading. It is frequently life threatening. Most often this complaint is respiratory or cardiac in origin, but can occur for other reasons such as pain, bleeding, or medication interaction/reaction. When assessing the patient, look for associated signs and symptoms. Is the patient experiencing shortness of breath cool, pale, and sweaty? Is there pedal edema? Does the patient have a history of respiratory illness? Is this similar to previous events? How is this time different?

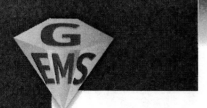

Section 2: Lectures

Slide Text	Additional Information
Slide #16 **Chief Complaint: Chest Pain** • Often cardiac in nature • **G:** Many experience pain differently. • **M:** Medication history is important. • Have the patient locate the pain. • Expose the chest: scars, pacemaker, medication patches	The complaint of chest pain is still most often associated with a cardiac event such as angina, or myocardial infarction. Aging affects how we sense pain (consider the "G" in the GEMS diamond). Many patients refer to chest discomfort or pressure or just an uncomfortable feeling. Use of an open question like "Tell me about the discomfort in your chest" may elicit a better response from the patient. Assessing the medications that the patient is taking may lead to clues to the patient's problem (consider the "M" in the GEMS diamond). A patient who takes nitroglycerin for angina and has not had relief from the same dose (unstable angina) may be progressing toward an MI. Location of the pain is important. Substernal pain may be cardiac, while pinpoint pain on the side of the chest wall can be just a pulled muscle. Look for scars on the chest that may indicate bypass surgery or pacemaker insertion. Also check for medication patches such as a long-acting nitroglycerin paste.
Slide #17 **Chief Complaint: Altered Mental Status** • Some causes manifest quickly, others over days • **M:** Medication reactions are a frequent issue. • Determine LOC and orientation to person, place, and time. • Check motor and sensory response. • **ALS:** Get an ECG and blood sugar reading.	Assessing the patient with altered mental status may require looking back over several hours or several days. Hypoglycemia may present over several hours while hyponatremia may be several days. Medication use or misuse can present as altered LOC (consider the "M" in the GEMS diamond). Determine the patient's level of consciousness and orientation. You will also need to determine the patient's norms here as well. Check motor and sensory response to assess for signs of stroke. **ALS:** Monitor the ECG, pulse oximetry, and blood glucose. All may lead to clues to the cause.

Section 2: Lectures

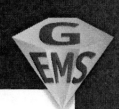

Slide Text	Additional Information
Slide #18 **Chief Complaint: Abdominal Pain** • **G:** More likely to be hospitalized • **G:** Potential causes change with age. • **G:** Overall pain response is decreased. • Patient history is key. • Look for additional signs.	An older patient with the complaint of abdominal pain is more likely to be hospitalized than his/her younger counterpart. Potential causes for the pain change with age. An older patient is less likely to present with appendicitis, but when it does occur the patient is sicker (consider the "G" in the GEMS diamond). The expected signs and symptoms may be altered or absent in the older patient. Older people typically have less abdominal pain perception and fewer related symptoms. A careful history with open-ended questions regarding the pain is important. Look for additional signs and symptoms such as tachycardia, tachypnea, or hypotension to help you determine the cause of the pain.
Slide #19 **Chief Complaint: Dizziness or Weakness** • Factors: balance, injury, oxygen, and energy • History will help clarify the complaint. • **ALS:** Check ECG, orthostatic changes, blood sugar. • Check for signs of stroke. • Assess for signs of head trauma.	A chief complaint of dizziness or general weakness can make it difficult to identify the cause. Factors to include in your assessment include balance problems from inner ear inflammation or infection, injury including stroke or head trauma, oxygen perfusion problems such as hypotension, hypertension, anemia, or arrhythmias. Glucose can affect the energy needed to effectively run the brain. History can help clarify the complaint. Dizziness means different things to different people. Assess for vertigo. Vertigo is most often a problem in the inner ear. Determine if the dizziness is at rest or with activity. Possible reasons for dizziness at rest include arrhythmias or severe hypotension. Dizziness with mild activity may indicate dehydration, anemia, or hypotension. **ALS:** Your physical assessment should include ECG monitoring, checking for orthostatic changes in blood pressure, and assessing the blood sugar. Check for signs of stroke. Use of an assessment tool like the Cincinnati Prehospital Stroke Scale can aid your diagnosis. Remember during your assessment to include questions regarding head injuries, even as far back as two weeks before.

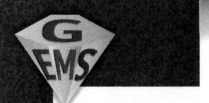

Section 2: Lectures

Slide Text	Additional Information
Slide #20 **Chief Complaint: Fever** • Normal response to infection • Suspect serious infection when accompanied by changed LOC. • Look for immediate life threats. • Fever means illness until proven otherwise.	Fever is the body's response to infection. When it is accompanied by decreased level of consciousness, you should suspect a serious infection. Look for life threats and treat them immediately. Fever means illness until proven otherwise.
Slide #21 **Chief Complaint: Trauma** • Exam follows the ABCs. • Look for potential medical causes. • Past history may change the needs of the patient. • Find the patient's baseline status. • G: Fractures are serious injuries.	With complaints of trauma the first things to assess are the ABCs. In the older population, the EMS provider must look for the underlying cause of the trauma. Did the patient have a stroke while driving and then crash his car? Did the patient get confused and walk into traffic? The treatment a patient needs may be altered based on their past medical history. A patient with COPD will require more frequent assessments and more aggressive treatment of trauma to the chest than another patient without the history. The assessment of the patient should look to determine the patient's historical baseline status. If a patient had a history of high blood pressure and it is now normal to low, aggressive therapy should be initiated. Fractures can be serious in older people (consider the "G" in the GEMS diamond). Fractures of a long bone can bleed significantly, producing shock in the hemodynamically challenged patient.
Slide #22 **Chief Complaint: Pain** • Unpleasant sensory or emotional experience • Use open-ended questions to evaluate. • Pain scale can be helpful. • Interpret vital sign changes as medical issues. • G: Older patients may hesitate to complain of pain.	Pain is defined as, "an unpleasant sensory and emotional experience associated with actual or potential tissue damage, or described in terms of such damage." Pain should be evaluated with the OPQRST mnemonic. Open ended questions will allow the patient to describe their "personal" experience. "Tell me about your pain" or "what makes the pain better or worse?" are good questions for evaluating pain. The use of a pain scale can also be helpful.

Section 2: Lectures

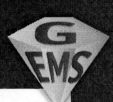

Slide Text	Additional Information
	Even though pain can be the cause of vital sign changes, the patient must be assessed for a medical cause. Pain may mask a potentially worse medical problem. Older patients often hesitate to complain of pain (consider the "G" in the GEMS diamond). Such concerns as, "My mother had a pain like this and she didn't make it," or fear of ending up in a nursing home may keep a patient from complaining of pain.
Slide #23 **Chief Complaint: Falls** • Generally result from contributing factors • Look for medical reason for fall. • Assess for injury and life threats. • **ALS:** ECG, blood glucose, pulse oximetry	The complaint of a fall is generally the result of contributing factors. Trips on loose rugs, dizziness from dehydration, or falling after a syncopal episode all result in injury from the fall, but the underlying cause is an additional concern. As a fall is a type of trauma, the trauma assessment, looking for life threats and injury, must be completed. Each fall should be evaluated for a medical cause. **ALS:** Assessing ECG, blood sugar, and pulse oximetry are a required part of the assessment.
Slide #24 **Chief Complaint: Nausea, Vomiting, and Diarrhea** • Can originate in or out of GI tract • **M:** Check for changes in diet or medications. • Look for signs of dehydration or electrolyte abnormalities. • Assess for GI bleeding.	Complaints of nausea, vomiting, or diarrhea can originate inside or out of the gastrointestinal (GI) tract. Check for changes in diet or medications (consider the "M" in the GEMS diamond). This will often be from GI-related illness. Look for signs of dehydration or electrolyte abnormalities. Peaked T-waves can indicate excess potassium. Assess these patients for signs of GI bleeding. Dark tarry stools or vomiting of coffee ground like material may indicate bleeding.

Section 2: Lectures

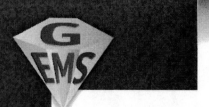

Slide Text	Additional Information
Slide #25 **Summary** • Changes with age affect assessment findings of older patients. • Emotional and psychological findings in the older patient should be evaluated. • Common complaints fall into ten main areas.	In order to better assess the older patient, the EMS provider must have knowledge of how the body changes with age. Slow or gradual changes are often the result of aging, while quick or sudden changes are often the result of illness or injury. Emotional or psychological findings most often are presentations of physical changes from illness or injury. Emotional or psychological changes in an older patient should be evaluated at a medical facility. The top ten common complaints were discussed. These will be the calls most often encountered by EMS.

Section 2: Lectures

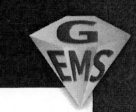

(BLS) Assessment of the Older Patient and Pharmacology

Teaching Tips

This lecture is specifically designed for a BLS audience. It covers assessment as well as pharmacology, since a medication history is an important part of the assessment of an older patient.

This lecture highlights the main points that are different in assessing an older patient. Be sure to emphasize that the assessment process does not change for an older patient. Students should still conduct the scene size-up, initial assessment, focused history and physical exam, detailed physical exam if applicable, and ongoing assessment.

This lecture also briefly discusses the top ten chief complaints of older patients, in order to familiarize students with the difficulties in determining the relationship between the complaint and the medical cause.

Be sure to tie-in the material from Lecture 2: Changes with Age, as it relates to the material presented here. This can be done with statements such as, "Remember that in Lecture 2, we learned that older people are more sensitive to temperature due to thinning of the skin and loss of fat."

Lecture Outline: Assessment of the Older Patient and Pharmacology

Slide Text	Additional Information
Slide #1 **Assessment of the Older Patient and Pharmacology**	This lecture covers topics found in Chapter 5: Assessment of the Older Patient and Chapter 13: Pharmacology and Medication Toxicity Emergencies.
Slide #2 **Objectives** • Describe normal and abnormal assessment findings. • Recognize common emotional and psychological reactions. • Describe common complaints in the older patient. • List the components of a medication history.	*Read objectives.*

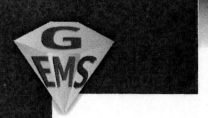

Section 2: Lectures

Slide Text	Additional Information

Slide #3
General Patient Assessment
- **E:** Scene size-up includes environmental assessment:
  - General appearance, cleanliness
  - Temperature, food
  - **S:** Drugs, alcohol, signs of abuse
- Initial assessment looks for life threats:
  - Airway cannot be protected as well.
  - Breathing can be complicated by previous disease.
  - Circulatory system has slowed responses.

Patient assessment follows the same format taught in your initial training. However, there are several factors that differ in assessing the older patient.

Scene size-up includes a thorough assessment of the environment. This is the "E" component of the GEMS diamond.

Look at the patient's general appearance. Can the patient dress, clean, and groom himself or herself without help? Does he or she have help if needed? This will begin to tell you how the patient manages their activities of daily living (ADLs). This is "S" in the GEMS diamond.

Pay attention to the temperature in the home. A cold home may indicate that the patient cannot afford to pay heating bills. Food is another indicator of how the patient manages financially. A lack of food will place the patient at risk for nutritional deficiencies.

Look around for signs of drugs, alcohol, or signs of abuse. Alcohol is a commonly abused substance for the older population. Signs of elder abuse may present as lack of care for the patient.

Initial assessment looks for life threats. These threats differ slightly in the older population. The airway is not protected as well as in younger people. Dentures, bridges, and other dental appliances can come loose and become an airway obstruction. The cilia that line the airway decrease in number, which allows easier aspiration of material.

Observing breathing can be complicated by previous disease. For example, a COPD patient would not be expected to have good chest rise with a barrel-shaped chest.

The circulatory system has slowed responses to stimuli. The older patient may have decreased pulses due to the changes in the vessels; the decreased pulse may not necessarily be due to the present illness.

Section 2: Lectures

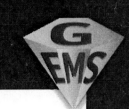

Slide Text	Additional Information
Slide #4 **Mental Status Assessment** • Confusion is not normal. • Distinguish chronic changes from new ones. • Enlist help from family. • Establish a baseline mental status. • Don't be misled.	During your assessment of the mental status, there are some things to remember. Confusion is not normal. Changes in mentation require additional assessment. Distinguish chronic changes from new changes. This can often be done with one question: "What is different today?" Enlist the help of family or caregivers. These are the people that know the patient's norms and can help you to determine the changes. Establish a baseline mental status. Changes in mentation are dynamic. You will often be called during an evolving episode. Be able to relate what your baseline was. Don't be misled. A patient who is showing early signs of dementia may try to divert your attention from your exam of his or her orientation. When asked about the day, his or her reply may be "Why should I have to know that!" The question was not answered and the provider may feel reluctant to ask again. Persist in your questioning in a kind but firm manner—it is important to address the pride and fear of the patient so that you obtain the needed information.
Slide #5 **Assessing the Chief Complaint** • Determining the chief complaint can be hard. • Start with what is bothering the patient most. • Chief complaints may not be the life threat. • Communication is a big component.	The chief complaint may be difficult to determine due to multiple disease processes or multiple complaints. It is often easier to ask the patient what is bothering him or her most or what is bothering him or her today. The chief complaint is not always the life threat. For example, pain from swollen feet may be fluid back up from CHF. Taking time to allow good communication between the caregiver and patient is a major part of assessment. Complaints may need to be examined one-by-one in order to determine the patient's condition.

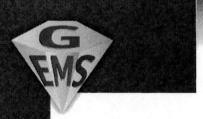

Section 2: Lectures

Slide Text	Additional Information
Slide #6 **Assessment** • Prioritize patient status. • Detailed physical exam • Ongoing assessment is required.	Before moving on with your assessment, you need to determine your patient's priority for transport. Table 5-1 lists several reasons why your patient may need rapid transportation. The detailed physical exam should be completed according to your patient's status. Unstable patients should have an exam done en route to the hospital, while less urgent patients should be examined before transport to minimize distractions. During your exam, issues related to thermal regulation may be a problem. Older patients will often wear multiple layers of clothing and when removed or opened up, they may become cold. Take measures to keep the patient comfortable while performing your exam; for example, only expose what you need to expose in order to perform your exam. Ongoing assessment is more important with older patients compared to their younger counterparts. Deterioration in the older patient's condition may be rapid. Vital signs should be taken every 15 minutes for a stable patient, while an unstable patient should have them taken every 5 minutes.
Slide #7 **Case Study 1** • Dispatched for an 82-year-old woman acting strangely; patient does not know why you are there. • Daughter states mother has Alzheimer's.	Your service is dispatched for a patient who is acting strangely. You begin to assess an 82 year-old woman, Mrs. Randish, who does not know why you are there. The daughter states that her mother has Alzheimer's disease and is acting strangely.
Slide #8 **Case Study 1 (continued)** • Daughter tells you that her mother is not listening today. • **G:** She tells you that her mother has had a cold.	The daughter continues by telling you that her mother is not listening today. She has asked her to do several tasks this morning, but her mother has not done any of them. She tells you that her mother has had a cold for a couple of days.

Section 2: Lectures

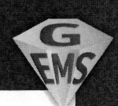

Slide Text	Additional Information
• **G:** Mrs. Randish is febrile, pale, and dry. *How would you approach the assessment of this patient?*	Mrs. Randish is febrile and her skin is pale and dry. Consider the "G" in the GEMS diamond, what might this presentation mean in an older patient. *How would you approach the assessment of this patient?* **(Elicit answers.)**
Slide #9 **Case Study 1 (continued)** • Pulse = 96 beats/min • Respirations = 24 breaths/min • BP = 110/70 mm Hg • Pulse Ox = 90% • Lungs have crackles in the lower left side. • Hands are cold.	Mrs. Randish's vital signs are a pulse of 96 beats/min, respirations of 24 breaths/min, a blood pressure of 110/70 mm Hg, and a pulse Ox of 90%. Lung sounds have crackles in the lower left lung. Her hands are cold.
Slide #10 **Case Study 1 (continued)** • Signs include increasing agitation per daughter. • Allergic to Sulfa • Medications include: Aricept, Paxil • Past history of Alzheimer's disease • Last meal was breakfast • Events are increasing agitation since this morning.	The case continues with a SAMPLE history. *Read slide.*
Slide #11 **Case Study 1 (continued)** • Mrs. Randish is becoming irritated with your questions. • Daughter is able to calm patient down. • Patient agrees to treatment and transport.	Mrs. Randish becomes irritated with your history taking and begins to talk loudly and act physically uptight. The daughter steps in and is able to calm the patient down. The patient agrees to be transported to the hospital.

Section 2: Lectures

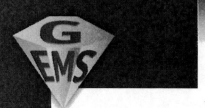

Slide Text	Additional Information
Slide #12 **Case Study 1 Conclusion** • Mrs. Randish is given oxygen to bring saturation into the mid 90's. • **ALS:** IV, cardiac monitor, 200 mL fluid bolus • She was transported to the hospital and diagnosed with pneumonia. • Mrs. Randish was treated and released after 1 week.	This case concludes with Mrs. Randish receiving oxygen, and IV fluids if an ALS unit is available. She was transported to the hospital and treated for pneumonia. The original complaint of "acting strangely" was not necessarily the patient's primary problem.
Slide #13 **Complaint-Based Assessment** • Relies on patient to clarify complaint • Requires in-depth verbal assessment • Complaints can be misleading. • Treat patient based on complaint and symptoms.	It is often useful to approach your assessment of the older patient starting with the complaint. This approach requires that the provider is able to communicate well with the patient and clarify the complaint. During the verbal assessment part of the exam, the complaint must be probed to determine the extent of the problem. Complaints can be misleading. A complaint of shortness of breath may be related to a cardiac cause, or a fall may have been precipitated by a episode of dizziness brought on by a cardiac arrhythmia. Treat these patients based on both their complaint and their symptoms. A patient with fever and a low blood pressure should be treated with oxygen and kept comfortable.
Slide #14 **Top Ten Complaints of Older People** • Shortness of breath • Chest pain • Altered mental status • Abdominal pain • Dizziness or weakness • Fever • Trauma • Generalized pain	The top ten complaints made by older people seeking medical care are listed on this slide. Some things to remember with each are: • Short of breath—often cardiac related • Chest pain—mostly cardiac but there are other causes • Altered mental status—look for causes including medication misuse, low blood sugar, stroke, or cardiac perfusion problems • Abdominal pain—can mask serious problems. All abdominal complaints must be evaluated in the ED.

Section 2: Lectures

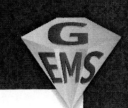

Slide Text	Additional Information
• Falls • Nausea, vomiting, diarrhea	• Dizziness or weakness—distinguish vertigo from dizziness and search for causes of dizziness. • Fever—usually due to infection. Assess for signs of shock. • Trauma—look for life threats, then look for medical reasons for the traumatic event • Generalized pain—older people sense pain differently as they age. • Falls—look for life threats, then look for medical reasons for the fall • Nausea, vomiting, diarrhea—assess for signs of dehydration.

Slide #15
Medication Assessment
• A comprehensive medication history is crucial.
• Barriers
  – Cognitive impairment
  – Underreporting
	In identifying drug-related problems, it is imperative to obtain a comprehensive medication history. The next slide will provide a map of how to assess an older person's medications.
	
	Barriers in the older patient can include cognitive impairment and underreporting. Cognitive barriers include forgetting what medications to take or when to take them. Underreporting occurs when a patient does not want to tell providers what medications he or she took.

Slide #16 **Medication History** • Prescribed medications • Adherence • Over-the-counter (OTC) medications • Herbal remedies • Other sources	Completing a medication history is an important part of the history of an older patient. Older people purchase as much as 25% of all prescribed medications and 33% of all over-the-counter medications sold in the U.S. The next slides will look at the components of the medication history.
Slide #17 **Prescribed medications** • Obtain a complete list, including doses. • Check prescribing doctor. • Look for new medications. • Ask about stopped medications.	When completing a medication history, list all of the medications that the patient is taking and their prescribed dosages. When copying the information from the medication containers, look for multiple prescribing physicians. Many patients have physicians for different problems. This can be a reason for polypharmacy.

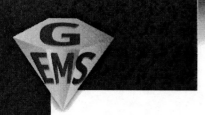

Section 2: Lectures

Slide Text	Additional Information
	Look for new medications or medications that have been recently stopped, as these may be reasons for common complaints.

Slide #18
Adherence to Prescription
• Determine if medications are taken as prescribed.
• Assess if medications are prescribed and not taken.
• OTC and herbal medications:
  – List all that are taken.
  – Determine why they are taken.
	Question the patient to see if the medications are taken as prescribed. Do they understand the instructions? Can they read them? Are there any medications that the patient is supposed to be taking but is not? This may happen because the patient cannot afford them or does not like the side effects.
	
	Many over-the-counter (OTC) medications can interfere with prescribed medications. Some of these are well known such as taking aspirin and warfarin (Coumadin); others are not as obvious. List all of the OTC and herbal remedies that the patient is taking in your history. Also try to determine why the patient is taking the remedy. It may be to control a side effect of one of the prescribed medications.

Slide #19 **Other Sources** • Has the patient taken another person's medications? • Is there evidence of alcohol or illicit drug usage?	The older patient may have access to many sources of drugs. A spouse, sibling, or child's medication may seem like it will help the problem. The patient may say, "It always works for my wife." Be astute during your environmental exam. Is there evidence of drug or alcohol usage? Alcohol is widely used in the older population and can affect other medications. An example is alcohol increasing the effects of a sedative such as alprazolam (Xanax).
Slide #20 **Case Study 2** • Dispatched to a residence for an uncontrollable epistaxis • 68-year-old woman, Mrs. Easton, found holding a blood-soaked towel	You are dispatched to a residence for an uncontrollable epistaxis. Upon arrival, you find an obese 68-year-old woman, Mrs. Easton, sitting on the sofa with her head back, holding her nose with a blood-soaked towel.
Slide #21 **Case Study 2 (continued)** • Uncontrollable nasal bleeding • BP = 210/160 mm Hg	Assessment reveals a conscious, alert patient with unmanaged, bright red bleeding from both nostrils. Mrs. Easton's face is flushed with petechial hemorrhages on the nose and cheeks. Vital signs

Section 2: Lectures

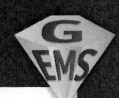

Slide Text	Additional Information
• Pulse = 136 beats/min • Respirations = 24 breaths/min	are a blood pressure of 210/160 mm Hg, a bounding pulse of 136 beats/min, and respirations of 24 breaths/min with effortless exchange.
Slide #22 **Case Study 2 (continued)** • Flushed skin • **G:** History of hypertension • **M:** Stopped medications because of cost	History: Mrs. Easton is under treatment for hypertension, but has not seen her physician for some time (consider the "G" in the GEMS diamond). She is prescribed diazoxide (Hyperstat), furosemide (Lasix), and potassium chloride (KCl). After some coaxing, Mrs. Easton explains that she could no longer afford the co-pay on the medications, and she felt really well, so she stopped taking them about two months ago (consider the "M" in the GEMS diamond).
Slide #23 **Case Study 2 Conclusion** • Medication nonadherence for economic reasons • **G:** Medications were changed to generic brands. • **M:** Mrs. Easton was enrolled in a prescription assistance program.	Mrs. Easton stopped taking her medication, and the cumulative effect is the current hypertensive crisis. The hypertension has probably elevated gradually since she stopped taking her medication, but since hypertension is completely insidious, she was not aware of her worsening condition. Mrs. Easton's medications were changed to generic prescriptions to assist her in maintaining adherence. She was also enrolled in a local prescription assistance program.
Slide #24 **Summary** • Changes with age affect assessment findings of older patients. • Emotional and psychological changes in the older patient should be evaluated. • Common complaints fall into ten main areas. • Medication history is an important part of assessment.	In order to better assess the older patient, the EMS provider must have knowledge of how the body changes with age. Slow or gradual changes are often the result of aging, while quick or sudden changes are often the result of illness or injury. Emotional or psychological changes most often are presentations of physical changes from illness or injury. Emotional or psychological changes in an older patient should be evaluated at a medical facility. The top ten common complaints were discussed. These will be the calls most often encountered by EMS. Completing a proper medication history can assist every level of healthcare provider that will deal with your patient in providing the correct care and eliminating potential medication problems later.

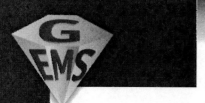

Section 2: Lectures

End-of-Life Care Issues

Teaching Tips

This lecture is brief but necessary to the course. While the procedures for handling patient death do not differ in the older population, the frequency of death will likely be greater on calls with this population. It is important that EMS providers understand how to handle patient death.

Because local protocols vary, it is critical that you customize this lecture to your area. Advance directives such as do not resuscitate orders (DNRs), living wills, and durable power of attorney are discussed, but specific guidelines regarding what is valid in your area are not given in this lecture outline or in the slide presentation. Verbally add information regarding local protocol as you are presenting this lecture. For example, you could ask students, "What is considered a valid DNR per our local protocol?" or "What would you do if a patient's relative supplied you with a living will? Would it be considered valid per local protocol? How would you be able to tell if it was valid?"

In preparation for this lecture, collect examples of DNRs and advance directives that are valid per your local protocol, as well as documents that would not be considered valid. Use these in the Scenarios portion of the course so that students can test their knowledge.

Lecture Outline: End-of-Life Care Issues

Slide Text	Additional Information
Slide #1 **End-of-Life Care Issues**	This lecture covers topics found in Chapter 4: End-of-Life Care Issues. *(This lecture requires modification based on your local protocol in order to be completely effective. Incorporate information and examples from your local protocol in order to give students concrete, practical information that they can use outside of the classroom.)*
Slide #2 **Objectives** • Discuss the principles involved in treating an older patient with a terminal disease. • Define palliative and hospice care programs. • Understand the legal ways for a patient to express his/her wishes at the end of life.	*Read objectives.*

Section 2: Lectures

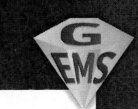

Slide Text	Additional Information
Slide #3 **Objectives (continued)** • Discuss grief and loss as they relate to the older patient, the family, caregiver, and EMS provider. • List the signs of impending death.	*Read objectives.*

Slide #4
End-of-Life Care
• Depends on patient's wishes
  – Some prefer aggressive resuscitative measures.
  – Others prefer palliative care only.
	The general goal of providing care to a patient with a terminal disease focuses on ensuring that the patient dies with dignity and is as comfortable as possible. Some patients may choose for EMS to provide aggressive resuscitative efforts, while others may prefer palliative care only. Although few people agree on what makes for a "good death," two common denominators include pain and symptom management and preparation for death, the latter being for the benefit of both the patient and the patient's family and friends.

Slide #5
Palliative Care and Hospice
• Palliative care
  – Active total care of patients whose disease is not curable
  – Provision of comfort measures only
• Medicare hospice benefit
  – Enables terminally ill patients to receive comprehensive end-of-life care
	In 1990, the World Health Organization (WHO) defined palliative care as "the active total care of patients whose disease is not responsive to curative therapy." It further identified the following components:
	• Affirming life and regarding dying as a normal process
	• Neither hastening death nor prolonging life
	• Provide relief from pain and other distressing symptoms
	• Integrating psychological and spiritual aspects of patient care
	• Offering support to help the family cope with the patient's illness and bereavement
	
	Hospice care can be provided in freestanding facilities, hospitals, nursing homes, or the patient's private residence. It is available 24 hours a day, 7 days a week. Hospice care can be provided by:
	• Family/caregiver
	• Patient's physician or hospice physician
	• Nurses and therapists
	• Clergy and social workers

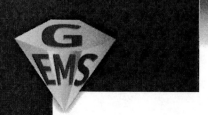

Section 2: Lectures

Slide Text	Additional Information
Slide #6 **DNR Orders** • If order is valid, CPR is not indicated for cardiac arrest. – Other invasive measures may be withheld as well. • DNR is only valid for the condition for which it is issued. • If validity is in question, begin BLS and contact medical control.	A "do not resuscitate" or DNR order is issued after the family and physician have discussed the "quality versus quantity" of life issue. This is carried out in a step-wise pattern. DNR does NOT mean do not treat! Other legal documents reflecting the patient's wishes were discussed earlier. Should the EMS provider have any question as to the validity of the DNR order, he/she should begin basic resuscitative measures and contact medical control for advice. It is important to note that if resuscitative measures are not taken, aggressive comfort measures are still needed: • Supplemental oxygen • Morphine or other narcotics for pain (if allowed per local or state protocol) • Placing the patient in a comfortable position DNR orders have been enacted in many states. If the document or device (commonly a wrist band) is valid, it should be honored. Usually, the DNR order means that if the patient develops cardiac arrest, CPR is not to be started. Other measures such as defibrillation, intubation, and other invasive therapies are withheld. Only supportive care is provided, such as non-invasive airway techniques and placing the patient in a comfortable position.

Slide #7
Advance Directives
 	
• Allow people to give directions about end-of-life care prior to its need
• Can be a:
  – DNR order
  – Durable power of attorney
  – Living will
	Advance directives are legal ways for a patient to express their wishes regarding health care at the end of life. They can be in one of three forms: a DNR order, a durable power of attorney, or a living will. The EMS provider must be familiar with all of these documents.
	
	The interpretation of various advance directives varies dramatically from state to state. It is important to consult your local protocols.

Section 2: Lectures

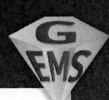

Slide Text	Additional Information
• Each state has laws regarding right to choose health care. Check protocols.	*(Discuss your local protocol here with students. Describe what is considered a valid DNR or advance directive per your local protocol.)*
Slide #8 **Durable Power of Attorney** • Appoints decision maker when patient is unable to make own health care decisions • Also referred to as health care proxies, health care agents • Appointed person makes decisions on patient's behalf and in accordance with patient's wishes	A durable power of attorney is a form of advance directive in which a patient appoints a person to make decisions regarding the patient's health care when they are unable to make decisions on their own. These documents are also referred to as health care proxies or health care agents. The appointed person makes decisions on the patient's behalf and in accordance with their wishes. *(Discuss your local protocol with regard to durable power of attorneys.)*
Slide #9 **Living Will** • Documents decisions regarding specific end-of-life treatments in particular situations • Typically more specific in terms of what care is to be provided • Also known as an instructional directive	A living will is another form of an advance directive. A living will documents decisions regarding specific end-of-life treatments in particular situations. In comparison to the durable power of attorney, the living will is typically more specific in terms of what care is to be provided. For this reason, the living will is also known as an instructional directive. *(Discuss your local protocol with regard to living wills.)*
Slide #10 **Case Study** • Dispatched to a residence for an 81-year-old woman, Mrs. Doe	Your service is dispatched for an 81-year-old woman, Mrs. Doe. The patient has entered a hospice program but has not yet been seen by the hospice care staff. The family called EMS because

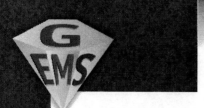

Section 2: Lectures

Slide Text	Additional Information
• Mrs. Doe just entered a hospice program but has not been seen. • Family called 9-1-1 because Mrs. Doe is gasping for air.	Mrs. Doe was found to be gasping for air. You note the address as you have responded many times for this patient over the past few years. The patient is in the end stages of emphysema.

Slide #11
Case Study (continued)
• Assessment reveals:
  – Gasping, irregular breaths
  – Skin cold to touch
  – Heart rate = 40 beats/min
	As you begin treatment, Mr. Doe hands you a document that he states is his wife's DNR order. He further tells you that his wife was adamant about dying in peace and with dignity. As you briefly glance at the document, the Doe's son arrives and confirms the legitimacy of the document. The husband asks that you take steps to make his wife comfortable, but without "heroics."

Slide #12 **Case Study (continued)** • Mrs. Doe is unconscious and unresponsive. • You hear a rattling sound when she breathes. • Airway is suctioned. • Family is asked if they want to be with her.	It is extremely important for EMS providers to recognize these signs of impending death and to provide comfort and reassurance to the family, communicating that this is part of the normal death cycle. Family members may or may not want to be with the patient during this time and you should facilitate their decision, whatever it may be. Other signs of impending death include: • Decreased food and fluid intake • Decreased urination (signaling shutdown of the renal system) • Increasingly more difficult to arouse • Decreased orientation • Decreased ability to see and hear • Irregular breathing patterns • Hypothermia or hyperthermia • Bradycardia or tachycardia
Slide #13 **Case Study Conclusion** • Mrs. Doe is now pulseless and apneic. • Per Mrs. Doe's and family's request, resuscitation is not initiated.	Once the patient has expired, your care must focus on the patient's family. At this point, comfort and reassurance that the patient did not suffer are very important.

Section 2: Lectures

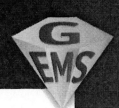

Slide Text	Additional Information
• You and your partner provide comfort measures for the family.	Prior to initiating conversation with the family, gather as much information as you can regarding the patient's death in order to convey a clear description. When possible, find a quiet room that is removed from the immediate area, which can sometimes be chaotic. When communicating with the family, you should use words such as "death" or "died." Euphemisms such as "passed away" should be avoided. You should be truthful with your responses to any questions. Offer to call a neighbor, other family member, or clergy, but respect the family's wishes if they do not want that. Older family members may have a particularly hard time dealing with the death of a loved one. If you as the EMS provider are finding difficulty in coping with the death of a patient, especially a patient that you knew personally, a critical incident stress management (CISM) process is in place in many organizations that serve EMS providers who deal with death and dying on a regular basis.

Slide #14
Summary
• Death is a part of life.
• EMS providers are faced with this on a regular basis.
• Support mechanisms must be in place to facilitate a healthy grieving process.
  – EMS support for family
  – CISM support for EMS provider
	One of the hardest things to do is to watch a patient die. In doing so, we must remember that death is a normal process of life. How we deal with the family and ourselves will make a significant difference in how we grieve.
	
	It must be recognized that the grieving process of denial, anger, bargaining, depression, and acceptance is normal and healthy, and will help the family resume a normal lifestyle. As EMS providers, we have a responsibility to the patient's family to facilitate this process by being there when needed.
	
	Let us not forget ourselves when dealing with the dead or dying. How we deal with the death of a patient can have a direct impact not only on our careers, but our psychological and physical health as well.

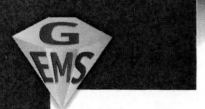

Section 2: Lectures

Trauma, Musculoskeletal Disorders, and Falls

Teaching Tips

Trauma is a major concern in the older population because it is more difficult for an older person's body to recover than for a younger person's body. It is important for students to understand the risks of trauma and falls in the older population, the impact of changes with age on their chance for recovery, and perhaps most importantly how immobilization techniques need to be adjusted to account for the older person's body. As in previous lectures, tie-in material from Lecture 2: Changes with Age throughout this lecture when applicable. For example, you could state, "Recall that in Lecture 2, we learned that an older person's reaction time is slower than that of a younger person. What injuries would you expect to see as a result of this?"

Make sure that the students understand that there are often underlying medical causes for trauma in an older person, and that they as EMS providers cannot strictly classify an older trauma patient as only a trauma patient. For example, the older fall patient may be both a trauma and a medical patient. It is important to fully investigate the cause of trauma in order to discover medical problems that may also require treatment.

Musculoskeletal disorders are not discussed in depth in this lecture, but it is a good idea to mention that they do exist and may make parts of the patient's body look disfigured. Students should keep this in mind when assessing for injury. The GEMS textbook contains further information on osteoporosis, osteoarthritis, and rheumatoid arthritis.

This lecture discusses immobilization concerns with the older patient, and this topic is covered in more depth in the corresponding video segment and skill station. Immediately following this lecture, show video Segment 3: Immobilization.

Lecture Outline: Trauma, Musculoskeletal Disorders, and Falls

Slide Text	Additional Information
Slide #1 **Trauma, Musculoskeletal Disorders, and Falls**	This lecture covers topics found in Chapter 7: Trauma and Musculoskeletal Disorders and Chapter 6: Falls.
Slide #2 **Objectives** • Discuss the epidemiology for trauma in older people. • Discuss the assessment findings in older patients with traumatic injuries. • Describe management and transport of the older trauma victim.	*Read objectives.*

Section 2: Lectures

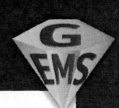

Slide Text	Additional Information
Slide #3 **Objectives (continued)** • Discuss the risk factors that make older people prone to falls. • Discuss essential components of assessing a fall. • Describe strategies used for prevention of falls.	*Read objectives.*

Slide #4
Injury Patterns
• Leading cause of death: falls, MVC, burns
  – Fewer MVCs, but with more severe injuries
  – Burns are associated with activities of daily living.
• Penetrating trauma is less common.
• Physical injury from elder abuse
	How injuries occur, the types of injuries, and the causes of injuries differ in the older adult. Falls are the leading cause of death, far outreaching all other causes combined. Motor vehicular trauma makes up the second cause, but these are on the rise. Pedestrian trauma is included in motor vehicular trauma. Burns are the third leading cause.
	
	The older population experiences fewer motor vehicle crashes than the rest of the population. However, when they do, it is with higher levels of injury. For example, airbags can cause greater injury to older patients, especially at higher speeds. The older population is involved in fewer accidents than most other age groups. Burn trauma is associated with activities of daily living (ADLs). Cooking, cleaning, smoking, or just moving past hot items are some of the causes of burns.
	
	Penetrating trauma is much less common in older people. A large number of the penetrating trauma deaths can be attributed to older men committing suicide. This is often done with a firearm.
	
	Physical injury from abuse is another form of traumatic injury (discussed in the Elder Abuse lecture).

Slide #5 **How Aging Affects Trauma** • Decreased pulmonary function and abilities • Hard to increase cardiac output	The key to understanding how trauma affects older people is in how the body changes with age. As we saw in Chapter 2, pulmonary function, or the ability to exchange gases, decreases. Also affected are the muscles used to move air in and out of the chest.

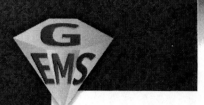

Section 2: Lectures

Slide Text	Additional Information
• Brain shrinkage allows bleeding. • Musculoskeletal system changes increase chance of injury.	Muscle mass decreases and the chest becomes less pliable, producing lessened ability to move additional amounts of air needed to compensate for trauma. Changes in the aging heart make it harder to increase the rate substantially, and for it to beat strongly. Atherosclerosis affects the body's ability to constrict the peripheral blood vessels, normally used to help compensate for blood loss. **ALS:** Remember that CO=HR x SV. Heart rate can be limited and an older heart cannot increase stroke volume well, therefore limiting how much cardiac output can be maintained. The brain will shrink with age. This shrinking causes the bridging veins between the brain and the dura mater to stretch. When the head sustains a sharp acceleration/deceleration motion, the bridging veins are torn and bleeding occurs. This bleeding can continue unobstructed until the cavity formed by the shrinkage is filled. Only then will the emergency provider encounter the common signs of increased ICP or Cushing's triad. Muscle becomes weaker with age. This can make the older person more prone to falls and makes less substance to cushion any impacts.
Slide #6 **Musculoskeletal Injuries** • Thoracic and lumbar spine injuries increase. • Upper extremities have high loss of function. • Less able to tolerate pelvic injuries – Hip fractures are debilitating and can be fatal. • Lower extremity fractures occur with less force.	In the category of musculoskeletal injuries, several areas stand out. The thoracic and lumbar spine experience more injury than that of a younger person. This is due partly to the loss of muscle supporting the structures, but also to the decrease in bone mass. These areas of the spine sustain a great deal of the vertical load of the body. When stressed, they are often injured. Upper extremity injuries are not often fatal. However, the use of the arms and hands is required for normal activities of daily living. The pelvis, like

Section 2: Lectures

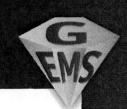

Slide Text	Additional Information
	other bones, becomes weaker. Fractures will bleed as quickly as in a younger person, but the older person does not tolerate blood loss nearly as well. Hip fractures can be immediately fatal or may begin a vicious cycle. This starts with the fall, then the patient decreases activity (especially those involving walking) for fear of falling again. This decrease includes activities normally needed to take care of oneself. Soon the body becomes weaker and an infection sets in (often pneumonia or UTI) and the patient has little ability to fight it. Lower extremity injuries occur with less force. This is due to less muscle to cushion the injury and the stresses encountered.
Slide #7 **ABCDEs for the Older Patient** • Airway: Dentures and lessened cough reflex • Breathing: Checking chest wall and respiratory drive • Circulation: Quality of pulses • Disability: Evaluating the patient's norms • Exposure: Modesty and hypothermia	Just as with trauma victims of other ages, assessment of the older trauma patient should begin with scene safety and ABCDEs. However, the ABCDEs for the older patient have their own unique pitfalls. Airway assessment must take into account any dentures or dental implants, crowns, or bridges. These can come out and produce an airway obstruction. Older patients also have a lessened cough reflex due to less cilia surrounding the airway. Patients may not be able to clear their own airway and aggressive suctioning is required. Also, C-spine stabilization should be attended to early due to higher incidents of C-spine trauma in older people. The breathing assessment should include an assessment of the chest wall and the musculature required to breath. Respiratory drive is another concern. Tidal volume and minute volume should be assessed early. Circulation assessment should include an early assessment of pulse quality. This will not only serve as a baseline but can give clues to hemodynamic status.

Section 2: Lectures

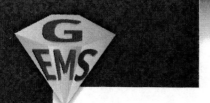

Slide Text	Additional Information
	Your disability assessment should take into account the patient's normal state. This can be hard to do unless someone who knows the patient is on scene. Exposure must include modesty and the risk of temperature imbalance.
Slide #8 **Assessment of the Older Trauma Patient** • Early baseline vitals • SAMPLE history • New pain or old • Physical exam • **M:** Must include medical evaluation	Although your trauma exam will not differ greatly from that of someone younger, several factors do need to be discussed. Because older patients do not compensate well for trauma, early baseline and constant repeat vitals will show the trends necessary to determine the patient's status. A SAMPLE history should be used to determine if the patient has past medical problems or is taking medications that may alter the physical exam or patient's response to trauma. Often, when asked about pain, the patient will list every pain that they are experiencing. When evaluating pain, the question of new pain or old pain must be asked. Physical exams must include what is normal for the patient. Older individuals have had a longer time to experience illness or injury leading to altered exam findings. An example would be a patient who has had a lung removed. Not knowing this could lead you to look for additional trauma that is not part of the problem. While the dispatch and current complaints are of a traumatic nature, you must take the time to evaluate any medical complaints that may have precipitated the trauma. Traumatic events are often just the consequence of a medical condition (consider the "M" in the GEMS diamond).

Section 2: Lectures

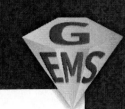

Slide Text	Additional Information

Slide #9
Considerations
• Conditions that may alter physical assessment:
  – Cataracts or asymmetrical pupils
  – Previous CNS condition
  – Previous surgeries
  – Decreased pain response
	Older patients often have conditions that may alter your physical exam. Cataracts or other conditions that can make the pupils asymmetrical may complicate your assessment of the pupils.
	
	Your exam can also be altered by conditions such as stroke or other CNS conditions that cause balance problems.
	
	Previous surgeries may alter the appearance of the patient or the function that is now normal for the patient.
	
	Decreased pain receptors throughout the body can alter the patient's ability to respond to pain. This is often the reason that older people sustain worse burns. After touching something hot, the decreased pain response does not register quickly enough and a burn has more time to generate.

Slide #10 **Management** • Treatment based on ABCs • Early spinal immobilization with padding • High-flow oxygen • Prevention of hypothermia • Rapid transport to appropriate center • **ALS:** IV access and cardiac monitoring	Treatment begins with supporting the ABCs. Early attention to spinal immobilization is necessary due to the unstable nature of older bone. Most older trauma patients will need substantial padding to make them fit onto a long spine board. Alternatives include the vacuum splint inflatable mattress, orthopaedic stretcher, or a blanket. Hypothermia is a potential consequence due to loss of subcutaneous fat and slower responses to regulate heat. Precautions must be taken to keep the patient warm. As with any trauma patient, early entry into the trauma system is paramount. Older people should be triaged even with lesser amounts of trauma due to their poor systemic response to trauma. **ALS**: IV access and cardiac monitoring are indicated for these patients. Fluid bolus amounts are controversial. It is believed that blood pressures should be kept near normal, however, patients with

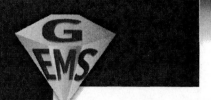

Section 2: Lectures

Slide Text	Additional Information
	hemodilution due to aggressive fluid replacement are another dilemma. Cautious volume replacement is indicated.
Slide #11 **Risk Factors for Falls and Injuries** • Sensory impairment • Brain diseases that affect balance • Dementia • Musculoskeletal disorders • Medications • Advanced age	Risk factors for falls include sensory impairment, especially related to eyesight and touch. Brain diseases, including stroke and Parkinson's, affect balance. Dementia influences balance and judgment and limits problem-solving abilities. Musculoskeletal disorders include osteoarthritis, rheumatoid arthritis, or previous trauma. Medications and medication reactions or interactions make falls more likely. Finally, age in and of itself is a risk factor.
Slide #12 **Assessing a Fall Patient** • Symptoms • Previous falls • Location of fall • Activity at time of fall • Time of fall • Trauma, both psychological and physical	Using the mnemonic SPLATT can be useful when assessing a fall. • Symptoms • Previous falls • Location of fall • Activity at time of fall • Time of fall • Trauma, both psychological and physical One of the best predictors of a fall is history of a previous fall. *Here, instructor can ask class to brainstorm on how to figure out when a patient fell if the patient does not know:* • Ask what patient was doing at time of fall. • Was sun out at time of fall? • If food is out, note what kind of food it is (breakfast food?) and ask patient what meal he/she was preparing. • Note what clothes the patient is wearing (pajamas) and ask if this is their normal attire for the current time of day.

Section 2: Lectures

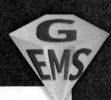

Slide Text	Additional Information
	Ask students why it is important to determine the time of the fall: • Pain may be due to being down for a long time. • Patient may have missed medications. • Patient may be hypothermic. • Patient may be dehydrated. • Pressure ulcers may have developed. • Greater chance of blood clots
Slide #13 **Preventing Falls in Older People** • Review of medications • Improvement of sensory function • Elimination of environmental obstacles • Strength and balance exercises	Prevention is something EMS should be involved in regularly. Some of the things that can be done to prevent falls include: • Take all of the patient's medications into the hospital so they can be evaluated for interactions • Increase the amount of light available. This can improve sensory function. Suggesting the use of a higher wattage light bulb or fixing a broken lamp may help prevent the situation the next time. • Eliminate loose rugs or extension cords that are on the floor or moving a hamper so the patient can get to the bathroom more easily. These are easy suggestions that can be made during the call. • Strength and balancing exercises are often needed to help the older patient maintain an active and healthy lifestyle.
Slide #14 **Case Study 1** • Dispatched to an MVC for a 75-year-old man, Mr. Sawyer, who drove into a tree • Moderate front end damage to car • E: Seatbelt and airbag used	You are dispatched to a one-car motor vehicle collision, car versus tree. You find a 75-year-old man, Mr. Sawyer, sitting behind the wheel of a mid-sized car that has impacted a tree. The car has moderate intrusion into the engine compartment. The air bag has been deployed and the patient has his seatbelt on (consider the "E" in the GEMS diamond). There is no other damage to the interior of the car.

77

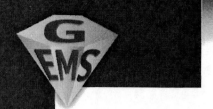

Section 2: Lectures

Slide Text	Additional Information
Slide #15 **Case Study 1 (continued)** • Mr. Sawyer complains of difficulty breathing. • Blood in mouth • Skin is pale. • He seems confused. *Where should your evaluation of Mr. Sawyer start?*	Mr. Sawyer is complaining of difficulty breathing. He states that he cannot catch his breath. He has a small amount of blood coming from his mouth and lip. His skin is pale and he appears confused about what happened. *Where should your evaluation of Mr. Sawyer start?* **(Elicit answers.)**
Slide #16 **Case Study 1 (continued)** • Labored breathing at 40 breaths/min • Lung sounds clear but shallow • Weak radial pulse of 88 beats/min • BP = 110/60 mm Hg • **ALS:** Pulse Ox = 92% • Tenderness to chest and abdomen	Mr. Sawyer is breathing at 40 breaths/min and has intercostal retractions. His lung sounds are clear but he is taking shallow breaths. He has a weak radial pulse of 88 beats/min. **ALS**: The monitor shows normal sinus rhythm without PVCs. BP is 110/60 mm Hg and pulse Ox is 92% on room air. He has tenderness to his anterior chest and abdomen with seatbelt marks beginning to show.
Slide #17 **Case Study 1 (continued)** • High-flow oxygen is applied • Mr. Sawyer is removed to a longboard. *Because of his kyphotic posture, Mr. Sawyer does not fit flat on the board. What can you do?*	High-flow oxygen is applied and Mr. Sawyer is rapidly removed to a long board. When you set him on the board, his head remains off the board and his shoulders rock from side to side. *Because of his kyphotic posture, Mr. Sawyer does not fit flat on the board. What can you do?* **(Elicit answers.)**
Slide #18 **Case Study 1 Conclusion** • Mr. Sawyer was immobilized and given high-flow oxygen. • Transported to trauma center • Diagnosed with a liver laceration • Died after two days in ICU	Mr. Sawyer received high-flow oxygen, proper immobilization, and **(ALS)** cardiac monitor and two large bore IVs. He was transported to the trauma center where he was taken directly to the OR. Mr. Sawyer was diagnosed with a liver laceration and pulmonary contusions. Mr. Sawyer developed acute respiratory distress syndrome (ARDS) and died after two days in the ICU.

Section 2: Lectures

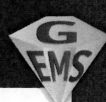

Slide Text	Additional Information
Slide #19 **Case Study 2** • Dispatched to 66-year-old woman, Mrs. Sozio, who fell in bathroom • Daughter found her on floor 6 hours after fall. • Mrs. Sozio complains of left hip pain.	You are dispatched to a residence for a 66-year-old fall victim. On arrival, you find an older woman, Mrs. Sozio, supine on the bathroom floor. The patient's daughter tells you that she found her mother here. Mrs. Sozio tells you that she fell around 6 hours prior to your arrival. Mrs. Sozio's complaint is of left hip pain. Her left foot is rotated inward.
Slide #20 **Case Study 2 (continued)** • Mrs. Sozio asks for glasses to see better. • E: You see a loose rug. • Your exam is hindered by an orthopaedic shoe on her left foot. *What were some of the risk factors that Mrs. Sozio had for falls?*	You notice Mrs. Sozio straining to look at you. You ask if she wears glasses and she asks you to get her glasses from the table. You notice a small throw rug on the floor (consider the "E" in the GEMS diamond). When trying to evaluate Mrs. Sozio, you notice an orthopaedic appliance on her left foot. *What were some of the risk factors that Mrs. Sozio had for falls?* **(Elicit answers.)** All three are risk factors.
Slide #21 **Case Study 2 Conclusion** • Mrs. Sozio is immobilized and transported to hospital. • Diagnosed with hip fracture • Returned home after rehabilitation	Mrs. Sozio had her hip immobilized and was transported to the ED for further evaluation and later surgery. She spent 1 week in the hospital and 8 weeks in a nursing home before returning home.
Slide #22 **Summary** • Top 3 causes of death: falls, MVC, burns • Assessment is modified for older patient. • Management includes maintaining ABCs. • There are risk factors that can predict a fall. • There are tools to assess falls. • EMS can prevent falls.	*Review slide.*

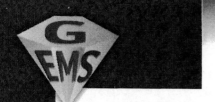

Section 2: Lectures

Neurological Emergencies and Altered Mental Status

Teaching Tips

Neurological emergencies are among the most complex aspects of geriatric emergency care. This lecture will introduce students to the importance of stroke recognition, determination of time of onset, and triage to an appropriate facility. It will also discuss the differences in delirium and dementia. Other neurological emergencies and conditions are also discussed throughout and treatment strategies are developed.

One way to improve synthesis of the information is to provide examples of a patient during the lecture, and ask if the students think the patient has delirium or dementia. This can be done once or twice using personal experience, or can be fictitious. For example, you could ask, "The patient has Alzheimer's but the daughter states that the patient has been acting strangely since this morning. Is it delirium or dementia? Consider this during the rest of the lecture—we will discuss it further throughout this lecture and in the Scenarios portions of the course."

You can also remind students that it is not as important as to identify the exact type of stroke as to identify that a stroke is occurring.

Lecture Outline: Neurological Emergencies and Altered Mental Status

Slide Text	Additional Information
Slide #1 Neurological Emergencies and Altered Mental Status	This lecture covers topics found in Chapter 10: Neurological Emergencies.
Slide #2 **Objectives** • Discuss abnormal changes with aging of the nervous system. • Discuss the epidemiology of nervous system disease in the older population. • Discuss assessment of complaints related to the nervous system. • Develop a treatment plan for complaints related to the nervous system.	*Read objectives.*
Slide #3 **Age-Related Changes in the Nervous System** • Be aware of normal changes in older patient's nervous system.	During the neurological examination of the older adult, the EMS provider must be aware of the normal changes that occur as a result of the aging process. Typically, these changes occur over an extended period of time and are usually not noticed by the patient's family. Neurologic diseases tend to

Section 2: Lectures

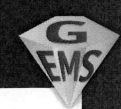

Slide Text	Additional Information
• Changes will affect neurologic examination: – Cognitive (thinking) – Speed – Memory • Postural stability	produce changes in neurologic function. This will result in a noted decrease in neurologic function. It is important to ascertain the patient's "baseline" mental status and neurologic abilities in order to determine if the problem is acute or chronic. The most frequent, normal changes in the older patient as the result of the aging process include: • Cognitive (thinking) ability decreases slowly with time. • Speed is affected in both the peripheral and central systems. • Memory has a slower retrieval time. This can make it difficult to obtain a reliable medical history unless family members are present to provide the information to you. Postural stability changes result in a high incidence of fall-related trauma.
Slide #4 **Causes of Altered Mental Status** • Can be difficult to determine in the older patient • Neurologic symptoms may be the result of multiple causes. • Use VITAMINS C & D mnemonic to recall potential causes.	A systematic approach to the neurologically impaired older patient will facilitate a field impression and subsequent management plan. The mnemonic "VITAMINS C & D" can be used to remember the more common causes of neurologic impairment.
Slide #5 **VITAMINS C & D** • **V**ascular • **I**nflammation • **T**oxins, trauma, tumors • **A**utoimmune • **M**etabolic • **I**nfection • **N**arcotics • **S**ystemic • **C**ongenital • **D**egenerative	*Discuss the components of the VITAMINS C & D mnemonic:* • **V** - Vascular: stroke, brain embolism • **I** - Inflammation: inflammation of the blood vessels in the brain (vasculitis) • **T** - Toxins: carbon monoxide poisoning; Trauma: concussion, intracerebral hemorrhage; Tumors: primary brain tumor, or **metastasis** (developed elsewhere and spread to the brain) • **A** - Autoimmune: production of immune system components against a normal structure in the central nervous system

Section 2: Lectures

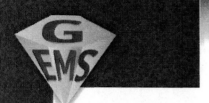

Slide Text	Additional Information
	• **M** - Metabolic: liver or renal failure, hypo/hyperglycemia, hypothyroidism, and nonketotic diabetes acidosis • **I** - Infection: meningitis, encephalitis • **N** - Narcotics and other drugs: there is a higher chance of these drugs causing a neurologic impairment if the patient has a pre-existing brain disease • **S** - Systemic: sepsis, hypoxia • **C** - Congenital: seizures • **D** - Degenerative: Alzheimer's disease and other dementias, Parkinson's disease

Slide #6
Stroke Facts
• Signs of stroke depend on type
  – Ischemic
  – Hemorrhagic
• Risk factors for stroke
  – Modifiable and preventable
	The signs of a stroke are dependant upon the type of stroke that the patient has suffered. Those with an embolic (clot) stroke (70–80% of all strokes) tend to present with the following signs:
	• Acute onset of mental confusion
	• Unilateral weakness or paralysis
	• Slurred speech (dysarthria)
	• Facial droop
	• Staggering gait (unable to walk without falling)
	
	The patient who is suspected of experiencing an ischemic stroke should be quickly evaluated, have their ABCs supported, and promptly transported to the hospital. Some patients with ischemic stroke are candidates for fibrinolytic (clot-busting) therapy if it is initiated within 3 hours after the onset of symptoms. The most important question to ask the patient's family is when the symptoms first appeared.
	
	Hemorrhagic strokes, which account for approximately 20–30% of all strokes, tend to produce the following signs:
	• Sudden, severe headache
	• Rapid loss of consciousness
	• Signs of increased intracranial pressure
	  – Cushing's triad
	  – Projectile vomiting

Section 2: Lectures

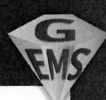

Slide Text	Additional Information
Slide #7 **Seizures** • Massive discharge of neurons in brain – Generalized motor seizures are most common. • Can be caused by many underlying factors	A seizure is a massive discharge of neurons in the brain. The generalized motor seizure (grand mal seizure) is most commonly encountered in adults and in older people. There are many underlying causes of a seizure, including cerebrovascular disease, brain tumors, drug ingestion, and head trauma. Initial care for the actively seizing patient is aimed at maintaining a patent airway and administering medications to halt the seizure.
Slide #8 **Dementia** • Brain disorder with memory impairment and loss of mental abilities with normal LOC • Multiple causes, including Alzheimer's disease • Gradual decline over many years	Dementia is a brain disorder characterized by memory impairment and loss of mental abilities but without a change in the level of consciousness. There are multiple causes of dementia including Alzheimer's disease, multi-infarct dementia (history of multiple strokes), nutritional deficiencies (Vitamin B12), chronic alcoholism, and tumors or other specific brain diseases. These patients experience a gradual decline of functioning leading to increased dependence on others for care in everyday activities. Psychiatric symptoms become more evident as the dementia progresses. Patients can become aggressive or depressive in later stages.
Slide #9 **Aggressive and Assaultive Behaviors** • Severe depression or dementia may cause aggression. • Aggression may be the result of fear or altered perception. • Provider safety is important.	Aggressive and/or assaultive behaviors may be seen in the older patient with severe depression or dementia. This may be seen because the brain disease has changed the patient's perception of their surroundings. Aggressive behaviors often come from the patient's internal fears. Calm reassurance can go a long way with these patients, however caregiver safety has to be the first concern. If the situation is unsafe, call for back up or police.

Slide #10
Delirium
• Acute rapid deterioration
• DELIRIUMS mnemonic may help in differentiating.
  • **D**rugs and toxins
  • **E**motional
	Delirium differs from dementia in one main fashion—it is usually reversible. Look for an acute onset of symptoms. This may progress over hours or a day or two. The mnemonic DELIRIUMS may be helpful in determining treatable causes of delirium.
	  • D—drugs and toxins
	  • E—emotional (psychiatric)

Section 2: Lectures

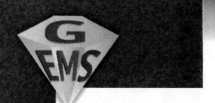

Slide Text	Additional Information
• Low PO$_2$ • Infection • Retention • Ictal • Under nutrition/dehydration • Metabolism • Subdural hematoma	• L—low PO$_2$ (COPD, CHF, AMI, pneumonia) • I—infection (pneumonia, UTI, sepsis) • R—retention (urine or stool) • I—ictal (seizure) • U—under nutrition/dehydration • M—metabolism (thyroid/endocrine, electrolytes, kidneys) • S—subdural hematoma

Slide #11
Parkinson's disease
• Loss of flexibility and fluidity in movement
• Decrease in the production of dopamine in brain
• Four cardinal signs:
  – Resting tremors
  – Rigidity
  – Slowness of movement
  – Postural instability
	Parkinsonism is characterized by a loss of flexibility and fluidity of posture and movement, combined with development of tremors usually seen in the hands. These symptoms are caused by decreased levels of dopamine. Parkinson's Disease is a type of Parkinsonism.
	
	In Parkinson's disease, there is a decrease in the production of the neurotransmitter dopamine.
	
	There are four cardinal signs of Parkinson's disease. Resting tremors (affect as many as 70% of patients), rigidity, slowness of movements (also called bradykinesia), and postural instability.
	
	There are other causes of Parkinsonism including carbon monoxide poisoning, multiple strokes, brain injury, and use of antipsychotic medications.

Slide #12 **Neurologic Assessment** • Begins immediately upon making patient contact – AVPU • Neurologic assessment of face • Neurologic assessment of extremities • Past medical history • History of trauma	The neurologic assessment of the patient begins as soon as you make patient contact. Using the AVPU scale, you can quickly determine the patient's level of consciousness. You should ascertain simple information by asking the patient if they know where and who they are. • Remember, due to the natural process of aging, the patient may not be aware of person, place, and time. This may be their baseline.

Section 2: Lectures

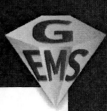

Slide Text	Additional Information
	Assess structures of the face, noting any facial droop, movement of the facial muscles in unison, or unequal pupils. The extremities should be assessed for equality of strength as well as sensory and motor function.
	The past medical history may yield key information as to what may be wrong with the patient. If the patient has a recent history of trauma (within 2 weeks) and an altered mental status, the cause of impairment is most likely structural damage to the brain and/or intracranial bleeding.

Slide #13
Stroke Evaluation
• Time of onset
• Cincinnati Prehospital Stroke Scale
  – Facial droop
  – Arm drift
  – Speech
• LA and NIH scales
	Stroke evaluation of the older patient starts with evaluation of the ABCs and additional life threats. The next step should be to determine the time of onset of symptoms. Therapies used in the treatment of stroke are time sensitive. Thrombolytic therapies need to be started within 3 hours from the onset of symptoms.
	
	The Cincinnati Prehospital Stroke Scale (see figure 10-3) is an easy assessment to confirm the presence of stroke like symptoms. The scale involves facial droop, arm drift (or weakness), and speech.
	
	There are other stroke scales that can be used as well. The Los Angeles Stroke Scale is a little more involved. The National Institute of Health Stroke Scale is very lengthy, making it not as optimal for use in the prehospital arena.

Slide #14
Patient Management
• For any patient with altered mental status, airway and ventilatory support have priority.
  – Supplemental oxygen at a minimum
  – Consider need for positive pressure ventilations.
• **ALS:** Monitor ECG, pulse Ox, and blood sugar.
	Regardless of the suspected cause of the altered mental status, support of the airway is of paramount importance. Many patients with altered levels of consciousness lose the reflexes necessary for spontaneous airway maintenance. This is especially true of the patient with a stroke.
	  • Manual positioning of the head (jaw-thrust if trauma is suspected)
	  • Insertion of an airway adjunct
	    – Remain alert for vomiting

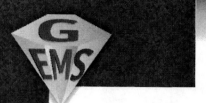

Section 2: Lectures

Slide Text	Additional Information
	• 100% supplemental oxygen if breathing adequately • Assisted ventilations if not breathing adequately – ALS assistance should be considered. The patient may require endotracheal intubation Because patients with neurologic dysfunction can deteriorate rapidly and with little warning, constant monitoring of vital functions (ABCs) is essential. The patient should be transported to the closest appropriate medical facility, with early notification of your status so that the most appropriate personnel and resources can be allocated. **ALS:** Patients should be monitored for ECG changes, Pulse oximetry, and blood sugar levels. Make appropriate changes in treatment to meet the needs of the patient.
Slide #15 **Seizure Considerations** • Continued airway support • Pad all hard objects near patient. • **ALS:** Administer an anticonvulsant. – Intravenously or via rectal route	Brief seizures are not usually problematic. Continued management of ABCs with oxygen and keeping the patient from further harm are the mainstays of seizure management. If it is determined that a patient is in status epilepticus, the EMS provider must act quickly or else the patient will die. Remember, seizure deaths are hypoxic deaths. Do not forget to check the patient's blood sugar level. Hypoglycemia, if detected early enough, can be easily reversed. The brain needs glucose as much as it needs oxygen. **ALS:** In addition to protecting the patient from injury and maintaining a patent airway with ventilatory support as needed, medications must be administered to halt the seizure. Benzodiazepine medications are used for this purpose: • Lorazepam (Ativan) • Diazepam (Valium) • Midazolam (Versed)

Section 2: Lectures

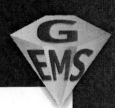

Slide Text	Additional Information
	Always adhere to local protocols regarding the administration of medications. Valium and Ativan can be administered via the intravenous (fastest). Valium can be administered by the rectal route if intravenous access cannot be obtained. Also, Versed is available by intramuscular (IM) injection.
Slide #16 **Case Study 1** • Dispatched to residence of 80-year-old Mrs. Casey, who is unconscious • Husband called, wife complained of sudden, severe headache	You are dispatched for an 80-year-old woman, Mrs. Casey, who is unconscious. The husband called EMS after his wife complained of a sudden, severe headache and then lost consciousness. The Casey's home is approximately 30 miles from the nearest appropriate medical facility.

Slide #17
Case Study 1 (continued)
• Assessment findings:
  – Unconsciousness
  – Rapid, irregular breathing
  – Hypertension
  – Bradycardia
• Therefore, signs of increased intracranial pressure (ICP)
• Husband says wife has a history of hypertension, denies trauma
	Mrs. Casey should be suspected of having an intracranial hemorrhage. Regardless of the cause, she is exhibiting signs of increased intracranial pressure and cerebral edema:
	• Unconsciousness
	• Rapid, irregular breathing
	• Hypertension and bradycardia
	  – The trio of hypertension, bradycardia, and altered respirations is referred to as "Cushing's Triad" and is a classic finding in patients with increased ICP.
	
	Other signs such as unequal pupils and projectile vomiting can be seen in patients with increased ICP.
	
	There are several pathologies that can result in increased ICP, such as hemorrhagic stroke, brain tumors/abscesses, and head trauma.
	
	Due to the absence of trauma and the history of hypertension, your index of suspicion should be very high for that of a hemorrhagic stroke.

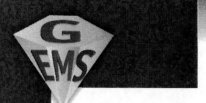

Section 2: Lectures

Slide Text	Additional Information
Slide #18 **Case Study 1 (continued)** • Mrs. Casey remains unconscious and her respirations are fast and irregular. • Your partner inserts an oral airway and initiates assisted ventilations. *What are the airway concerns with this patient?*	Since Mrs. Casey is unconscious, she cannot control her own airway; therefore, an airway adjunct must be inserted. Additionally, her breathing is inadequate and must be managed with assisted ventilations (positive pressure ventilation). If ALS is not present, the BLS provider should consider requesting them. Paramedics can provide more definitive airway control (ie, endotracheal intubation). *What are the airway concerns with this patient?* **(Elicit answers.)** Specific concerns for Mrs. Casey include the potential for projectile vomiting, which increases the risk of aspiration and potential cardiac arrest.
Slide #19 **Case Study 1 Conclusion** • Mrs. Casey is placed on stretcher in a head-high position and rapidly transported to hospital. • Upon arrival, she is diagnosed with a hemorrhagic stroke.	After initial management of vital functions at the scene, the patient is rapidly transported to the hospital where a CT scan confirms a large intracerebral hemorrhage. Mrs. Casey is stabilized in the emergency department and taken to the operating room where the hemorrhage is repaired. She recovers from the surgery but has some residual neurologic impairment.
Slide # 20 **Case Study 2** • Dispatched to 70-year-old Mr. Neves, who is actively seizing • Per family, he has no history of seizures, recently diagnosed with a brain tumor • Family did not witness onset of seizure	You receive a call for a 70-year-old man, Mr. Neves, who is actively seizing. Mr. Neves' family denies any history of seizures. Mr. Neves has recently been diagnosed with a brain tumor. Although tumors and the pressure that they can place on structures in the brain can easily cause a seizure, they are not the only cause of seizures. Other causes must be considered.

Slide #21
Case Study 2 (continued)
• Upon your arrival, Mr. Neves' seizure has stopped.
  – He is unresponsive.
  – Pupils are unequal.
  – Respirations = shallow at 28 breaths/min
  – Heart rate = 130 beats/min
	Mr. Neves is showing abnormal neurologic signs despite the fact that the seizure has stopped. Seizures typically produce a postictal state immediately after the seizure, however, the patient gradually recovers over time. The findings with this particular patient suggest an underlying neurologic pathology. The seizure could be the result of the expanding tumor or an intracerebral hemorrhage.

Section 2: Lectures

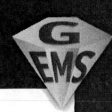

Slide Text	Additional Information
What is the initial management for this patient?	*What is the initial management for this patient?* **(Elicit answers.)** Initial management for Mr. Neves should focus on supporting his respirations with positive pressure ventilations and being alert for vomiting.
Slide #22 **Case Study 2 (continued)** • Mr. Neves is still unconscious. • Begins having another seizure • Becomes cyanotic during seizure *What is happening to Mr. Neves?*	Since Mr. Neves did not regain consciousness in between seizures, he is experiencing status epilepticus. Status epilepticus is defined as a prolonged seizure or when two or more seizures occur without a return of consciousness in between the seizures. Status epilepticus is a true life-threatening condition that requires immediate intervention and rapid transport. *What is happening to this patient?* **(Elicit answers.)** Mr. Neves is becoming severely hypoxic due to the repeated seizures.
Slide #23 **Case Study 2 (continued)** • Mr. Neves is fully immobilized and transported. • **ALS:** Intravenous diazepam (Valium) administered – Seizure stops after 5 mg of diazepam. • **ALS:** Blood glucose level checked en route.	Due to the fact that the family did not witness the onset of the seizure, trauma cannot be ruled out. Therefore, Mr. Neves must be immobilized as though a spinal injury exists. **ALS:** Following the administration of 5 mg of Valium, Mr. Neves' seizure stops. Rapid transport is continued to the hospital with airway support continued en route. The patient's blood glucose level is 110 mg/dL. Remember, if any possibility of trauma exists, err on the side of full spinal immobilization.

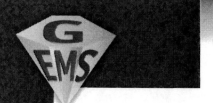

Section 2: Lectures

Slide Text	Additional Information
Slide #24 **Case Study 2 Conclusion** • At hospital, CT reveals a large tumor in occipital lobe of brain. – When compared to a prior CT, tumor has grown significantly. • Other neurologic diseases are ruled out.	It has been determined that Mr. Neves' brain tumor was the cause of the seizure. Clearly, it has grown large enough to put pressure on the brain. Its location in the occipital lobe would explain the unequal pupils. Other neurologic diseases that could have caused this seizure include: • Meningitis • Encephalitis • Encephalopathy • Any degenerative disease of the brain
Slide #25 **Summary** • Alterations in mental status can have many causes. • VITAMINS C & D is an effective tool to attempt to identify underlying cause. • EMS provider's main role is to support ABCs and transport promptly.	Because there are so many causes of an altered mental status, it is not beneficial to the patient to waste time in the field attempting to determine the underlying etiology. Abnormalities that can be quickly fixed (ie, hypoglycemia) must be treated immediately upon discovery. The mainstays of management are support of airway, breathing, and circulatory function and immediate transport for diagnosis and definitive care. Remember that older adults may present with abnormal neurologic findings that are "baseline" for them. You must determine what has changed and in what way. Acute abnormal neurologic signs can be the result of more than one problem. Do not assume that the patient's problem is isolated.

Section 2: Lectures

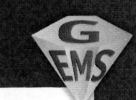

Respiratory and Cardiovascular Emergencies

Teaching Tips

Respiratory and cardiovascular emergencies are some of the most common emergencies in the older population. While treatment may not vary for these emergencies, the frequency in the older population warrants a good refresher of the material.

As taught in Lecture 2: Changes with Age, the signs of a cardiovascular emergency may be different in an older patient. Tie-in the material from that lecture, where applicable, to improve student's retention of that knowledge.

Consider telling students about personal experiences you may have had with these types of emergencies, and providing tricks of the trade that can be used when identifying problems and treating these patients.

Lecture Outline: Respiratory and Cardiovascular Emergencies

Slide Text	Additional Information
Slide #1 **Respiratory and Cardiovascular Emergencies**	This lecture covers topics found in Chapter 8: Respiratory Emergencies and Chapter 9: Cardiovascular Emergencies.
Slide #2 **Objectives** • Discuss the epidemiology of pulmonary and cardiac diseases in the older population. • Compare and contrast the pathophysiology of pulmonary and cardiac diseases with those of younger adults. • Be able to identify the need for treatment and transport for older patients with pulmonary and cardiac complaints.	*Read objectives.*
Slide #3 **Respiratory Issues Related to Aging** • Physiologic reserves are decreased. • History of underlying disease • Respiratory assessment can be challenging. • **M:** Medications can complicate the situation.	As we age, there are several issues that alter the way the body reacts to respiratory compromise. In general, physiologic reserves are decreased with age. The body no longer has the ability to increase the oxygen intake in response to illness or injury.

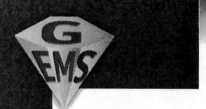

Section 2: Lectures

Slide Text	Additional Information
	Older adults often have a history of previous disease. Damage from an episode of pneumonia can complicate the body's ability to overcome another episode. Respiratory assessment can be complicated when there are atypical presentations or when symptoms overlap in their presentation. It may be hard to separate a CHF patient who is having difficulty when stricken by pneumonia. Medications often complicate the assessment (consider the "M" in the GEMS diamond).
Slide #4 **Assessment of Respiratory Complaints** • History may suggest the problem. • SAMPLE history should be completed. • Some questions to ask include: – Have you ever had this before? – How many pillows do you sleep on? – Have you changed any of your medications?	Older people are a great source of information. Many times they have been through an episode of something prior to the current one. In getting a SAMPLE history, they will often tell you what is affecting them this time. Some additional questions that can help to narrow down the possibilities include: 1. Have you ever had this before? While an answer of "yes" doesn't mean that it is the same thing again, it is very likely. 2. How many pillows do you sleep on? This can help to determine if the patient suffers from orthopnea, or increased trouble breathing when lying flat. Commonly this is associated with CHF. 3. Have you changed any of your medications? Medication side effects can precipitate respiratory complaints. An example would be beta-blocker eye drops (timolol), which can trigger asthma in some patients.
Slide #5 **Components of a Respiratory Exam** • Inspection • Palpation • Percussion • Auscultation	Examination of the chest during a respiratory exam includes four steps: inspection, palpation, percussion, and auscultation. Inspection includes looking at the pattern of breathing and movement and symmetry of the chest wall. Cyanosis or pallor may be seen in low oxygen states. Check for accessory muscle usage as well.

Section 2: Lectures

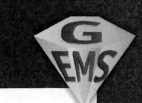

Slide Text	Additional Information
	Palpate to check for chest wall tenderness and asymmetrical motion. Vibrations from secretions in the airways can also be felt.
	Percussion is a tool not often used in the field due to the high ambient noise. However, this is a useful tool in a quieter setting.
	Auscultation is a normal part of our exam. Abnormal airway sounds include: wheezes, crackles, rhonchi, stridor, and even a pleural friction rub. This part of the exam often sets the tone for our continued treatment.
Slide #6 **Chronic Obstructive Pulmonary Disease (COPD)** • Asthma • Emphysema • Chronic bronchitis	Chronic obstructive pulmonary disease, or COPD, has multiple forms. Asthma is a disease characterized by bronchospasm, edema of the lining of the airways, and accumulation of secretions, and may be triggered by viral infections, air pollutants, allergens, or medications. Examination may reveal inspiratory and expiratory wheezing and a prolonged expiratory phase. Emphysema produces lung destruction that leads to progressive dyspnea. It is frequently caused by cigarette usage. Chronic bronchitis has an associated cough and sputum component that is prominent in the morning.
Slide #7 **Pneumonia** • Major killer of older adults • Presentation may differ in older people. • Crackles, pus in sputum, fever, loss of appetite	Pneumonia is the fifth leading cause of death in the older population. The patient presentation is often different than that of a younger adult. Fever and a sputum-producing cough are common in the younger patient, but an older patient may not experience fever and the cough can be negligible due to dehydration. Other common signs include crackles (common to the affected section of lung), loss of appetite, and fatigue.

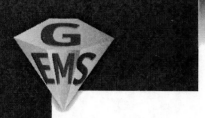

Section 2: Lectures

Slide Text	Additional Information
Slide #8 **General Emergency Respiratory Management** • Reduce patient's anxiety by reassurance. • Protect the airway. • Allow position of comfort if patient can maintain. • Oxygen is indicated. • If patient has an inhaler, assist patient with a dose. • ALS: Other medications as situation warrants within local protocol.	Care for respiratory management starts with trying to reduce the patient's anxiety. Protect the airway, but allow the patient to remain in his or her position of comfort if possible. To force them into a position that is unnatural will only increase the stress and increase the anxiety level. Oxygen should be delivered to the patient as needed. Saturations monitored by pulse Ox should be in the mid 90s. If the patient has an inhaler, providers can assist the patient in using it. ALS treatment should be geared at managing the cause of the distress. Bronchodilators for bronchoconstriction, diuretics for fluid build up.
Slide #9 **Cardiovascular Disease** • Most common cause of death in older people • CAD and CHF top the list. • Dyspnea is often the complaint. *How should you begin to differentiate cardiac from respiratory causes?*	Diseases of the heart are listed as the number one killer of older people. Coronary artery disease (CAD) and congestive heart failure (CHF) are the leaders in this category. Because atypical disease presentations are common in older people, dyspnea is the most often-heard complaint with cardiac-related causes. *How should you begin to differentiate cardiac from respiratory causes?* **(Elicit answers.)**
Slide #10 **Taking a History** • **G:** Compare signs and symptoms to previous events. • Past diagnoses are a good place to start. • **M:** Medications may lead you to a cause. • Compare events leading up to today with patient's normal activity.	History is very important in determining the cause of the event. During your history taking, try to compare signs and symptoms with previous events. This will allow the patient to describe how this event is similar to or different from a previously diagnosed problem. If an individual tells you that his chest pain is just like his previous MI, it is a good bet that this is another one (consider the "G" in the GEMS diamond). A good medical detective looks at the medications to determine what kind of medical history the patient may be suffering from (consider the "M" in the GEMS diamond). Someone who takes medications related to controlling hypertension may have other cardiac problems also.

Section 2: Lectures

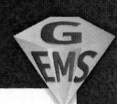

Slide Text	Additional Information
	Compare the events that led up to the event today with the patient's normal activity. If a patient can normally walk up the stairs without getting winded, but today they are short of breath, that shows something new.
Slide #11 **Clinical Presentation of Angina or AMI** • May experience no pain or atypical pain • Less localized, vague, not "crushing" or "squeezing" • Dyspnea, fatigue, syncope, nausea, confusion • Palpitations upon effort or sweating • Ask about discomfort, not pain.	The classical presentation of substernal chest pain with radiated pains down the left arm may not be present in the older patient experiencing cardiac-related pain. Many older patients may experience no pain from angina or acute myocardial infarction (AMI). Those who do often have a less localized pain that is not "crushing or squeezing" as is taught in initial training. Dyspnea, fatigue, syncope, nausea with or without vomiting, or confusion all can be symptoms of a cardiac event. Palpitations with exertion or sweating without exertion can also indicate a cardiac-related event. When questioning the older patient about chest pain, it is often better to use the term "discomfort," as they may not feel "pain" in the classic sense.
Slide #12 **Management of Angina and AMI** • Decrease anxiety, make patient comfortable • Maintain ABCs, high-flow oxygen. • Nitroglycerin q 5 min • **ALS:** IV, monitor, 12-lead ECG, consider aspirin, morphine • **ALS:** If hypotension develops, place in modified Trendelenburg's, give 250 mL bolus crystalloid.	Treatment of the suspected AMI does not differ greatly from a young adult to an older adult. Care should be used to make the patient comfortable, thereby decreasing stress to the heart. Maintain the ABCs and be ready to intervene if necessary. High-flow oxygen is required. Administer additional nitroglycerin as protocol allows and begin transport. Note: Nitroglycerin may act synergistically with many of the antihypertensive agents in older adults. This may cause the blood pressure to drop quickly. If this happens, place the patient in the modified Trendelenburg's position and give a 250 mL bolus of crystalloid. **ALS:** Establish an IV line at a TKO rate, cardiac monitor, and 12-lead ECG if available. Medication should include nitroglycerin 0.4 mg sublingually every 3–5 minutes. Consider aspirin or morphine sulfate if these are available.

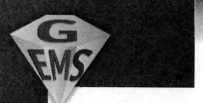

Section 2: Lectures

Slide Text	Additional Information
Slide #13 **Thrombolytic/Fibrinolytic Therapy** • Age is not a contraindication. • When did the pain begin? • Are there any bleeding disorders? • Brain cancer/masses or stroke? • On blood thinners? • Any recent surgery?	Thrombolytic and fibrinolytic therapy is indicated in many patients experiencing AMI. Age is not a contraindication for thrombolytic therapy. Patients up to 75 years old are treated in a similar fashion to the younger population. Above age 75, it is still considered an acceptable, safe, and useful intervention. There are several questions to help the ED staff decide if there are contraindications. Time is of the essence. These should be given no later than 6 hours from the onset of the symptoms. The therapy will dissolve clots. If the patient does not clot well already, they can bleed to death. Trauma or lesions in the brain may precipitate another stroke.
Slide #14 **Management of CHF** • Keep patient upright to allow fluid shunting. • Maintain ABCs. • High-flow oxygen • CPAP or BiPAP can be a useful tool. • **ALS:** IV, ECG monitor, advanced airway if needed, 12-lead ECG • **ALS:** Medications: nitroglycerin, furosemide (Lasix), morphine, and aspirin if chest pain is present	Management of CHF includes keeping the patient upright. This can allow the fluid to shunt toward the bottom of the lungs. Stretchers and carrying devices that require the patient to lay flat should not be used as the fluid may choke off airflow. The ABCs must be maintained. If the patient cannot maintain his or her own airway, ALS or rapid transport is required. Oxygen should be administered by a partial nonrebreathing mask or by bag-valve-mask connected to oxygen and a reservoir. Continuous positive air pressure (CPAP) or bilevel continuous positive airway pressure (BiPAP) can be a useful tool in the treatment of CHF. Many EMS systems are successfully using CPAP or BiPAP to decrease the number of patients who require intubation. There are no contraindications in the older population. **ALS:** IV at a TKO rate, cardiac monitor, and airway control if indicated should be assured. A 12-lead

Section 2: Lectures

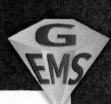

Slide Text	Additional Information
	ECG is helpful if the time and personnel needs allow. Medications that may be useful for this patient are included in the mnemonic MONA. Morphine, oxygen, nitroglycerin, and if the patient is experiencing chest pain, aspirin.
Slide #15 **Arrhythmias** • Many types affect the older population. • Atrial fibrillation is common. • Control of ABCs • Rate control if rapid ventricular response • 12-lead ECG is helpful.	There are many arrhythmias that affect older people. Atrial fibrillation is commonly found in this population and will be the only one discussed separately. As we age, the number of pacemaker cells in the sinus node (where normal sinus rhythms start) decreases, allowing other cells to take over. The rate of discharge in A-fib can exceed 300–500 times per minute. The ventricles cannot handle this fast pace and do not keep up. However, when the ventricular response increases, rate control is indicated. A 12-lead ECG is helpful in making the diagnosis of A-fib.
Slide #16 **Hypertension** • Affected organs: heart, eyes, brain, kidneys • Pressure should be lowered slowly. • A quick drop can result in stroke, AMI, or death. • **ALS:** Beta-blockers, sodium nitroprusside, or IV nitroglycerin	Hypertension is the last of the cardiac emergencies that we will discuss. Hypertension affects end organ perfusion. Some of the organs commonly affected are the heart, eyes, brain, and kidneys. Signs that someone's blood pressure has risen too high include pain or alterations of function of the end organs. This pressure will be different for every patient so it is hard to set a specific BP that indicates hypertension. **ALS:** When present, hypertension should be treated cautiously. Blood pressure should be lowered slowly. Common medications available to some ALS systems include beta-blockers such as labetolol, sodium nitroprusside, or IV nitro. If the pressure is allowed to drop too quickly, the patient can experience stroke, AMI, or death.
Slide #17 **Case Study 1** • Dispatched for 92-year-old Mr. Laube with difficulty breathing • Has COPD and makes frequent calls to EMS • Was intubated last time you responded	You are dispatched for a 92-year-old man, Mr. Laube, with difficulty breathing. Your partner says, "I remember that address. He is a bad COPD'er. The last time I was there we had to intubate him."

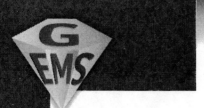

Section 2: Lectures

Slide Text	Additional Information

Slide #18
Case Study 1 (continued)
• When you enter, Mr. Laube is in the tripod position.
• Has intercostal and suprasternal retractions
• Speaks in broken sentences
• Vital signs:
  – Pulse = 104 beats/min
  – Respirations = 40 breaths/min
  – Blood pressure = 142/96 mm Hg
  – Pulse Ox = 86%
	When you enter Mr. Laube's house, you find him sitting in a chair tripoding. He has obvious intercostal and suprasternal retractions, and is speaking in broken sentences. His pulse is 104 beats/min, respirations 40 breaths/min, BP 142/96 mm Hg, pulse Ox 86% on room air, and the ECG shows sinus tachycardia.
	
	Ask class what other information would help in this assessment.
	(Elicit answers.)

Slide #19 **Case Study 1 (continued)** • Mr. Laube states, "This is the same as the other times." • **M:** Medications include his inhalers and a steroid. • You hear tight inspiratory and expiratory wheezes. *What are some of the other pulmonary diseases that affect older patients?* *How should you manage Mr. Laube?*	Mr. Laube states, "This is the same as the other times," referring to previous episodes of respiratory distress. He has tried his inhaler but said it did not help. As fast as he is breathing, you are not sure if he used the MDI correctly. He has two inhalers, beclomethasone (Vanceril) and albuterol (Proventil), and is taking a steroid (consider the "M" in the GEMS diamond). Listening to his chest, you hear a very tight monotone inspiratory and expiratory wheeze. *What are some of the other pulmonary diseases that affect older patients?* *(Elicit answers.)* COPD, pneumonia, pulmonary embolism, and pulmonary edema (CHF) are among the common types. *How should you manage Mr. Laube?* *(Elicit answers.)* *Discuss local management protocols.*

Section 2: Lectures

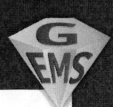

Slide Text	Additional Information
Slide #20 **Case Study 1 Conclusion** • Patient allowed to remain in tripod position. • Oxygen administered • **ALS:** 2.5 mg nebulized Proventil started • **ALS:** IV established at KVO rate. • **ALS:** En route, Mr. Laube received 2nd treatment. • Treated for exacerbation of COPD, but died later that night	Mr. Laube was allowed to remain in a position of comfort as transport needs allowed. High-flow oxygen was administered. Note: Administering high-flow oxygen over a long period of time can harm or kill patients with COPD, who may lose their respiratory drive when over oxygenated. Be aware of this and consider administering oxygen at a lower rate for these patients if local protocol allows. Mr. Laube is assisted in using his inhaler, then transported to the hospital. **ALS:** IV of normal saline (NSS) was established at a keep-the-vein-open (KVO) rate. 2.5 mg of Proventil by nebulizer was started and the patient was given a second dose en route to the hospital. Mr. Laube was treated in the ED for exacerbation of COPD, but died later that night.
Slide #21 **Case Study 2** • 67-year-old Mrs. Saunders has difficulty breathing • Rate = 30 breaths/min, slight retractions • Pale, sweaty, cool to touch; denies chest pain or other cardiac symptoms	You arrive at a house to find a 67-year-old woman, Mrs. Saunders, complaining of difficulty breathing. She is breathing at 30 breaths/min with slight intercostal retractions. She is pale, cool, and clammy. She denies chest pain, nausea/vomiting, or other cardiac-related symptoms.
Slide #22 **Case Study 2 (continued)** • Mrs. Saunders states she feels like this when fluid builds up. • **M:** Takes furosemide (Lasix), digoxin (Digatek), and potassium (K-Dur) for CHF • **G:** Has a history of CHF, A-fib, and AMI *Are all respiratory complaints caused by respiratory diseases?*	Mrs. Saunders tells you that this is the way she feels when her lungs fill with fluid. She is on furosemide (Lasix), digoxin (Digatek), and potassium (K-Dur) (consider the "M" in the GEMS diamond). She has a history of CHF, atrial fibrillation, and an acute myocardial infarction 4 years ago (consider the "G" in the GEMS diamond). She has taken all of her medications today as usual. *Are all respiratory complaints caused by respiratory diseases?* **(Elicit answers.)** No. There are many causes of respiratory distress in the older patient.

Section 2: Lectures

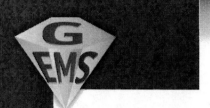

Slide Text	Additional Information
Slide #23 **Case Study 2 (continued)** • Pulse = 120 beats/min • Respirations = 30 breaths/min • BP = 190/100 mm Hg • Pulse Ox = 88% • Crackles • JVD, pedal edema bilaterally *How should you manage Mrs. Saunders?*	Mrs. Saunders' pulse is 120 beats/min, respirations are 30 breaths/min, BP is 190/100 mm Hg, pulse Ox is 88%, and the ECG is A-fib. Crackles are heard 1/3 of the way up her back. She has JVD and pitting edema of the ankles +2 bilaterally. *How should you manage Mrs. Saunders?* **(Elicit answers.)** **Discuss local management protocols.**

Slide #24
Case Study 2 Conclusion
• Patient seated upright on cot with high-flow oxygen
• Delivered to waiting cardiac team
• ALS:
  – IV, ECG, nitroglycerin × 3, furosemide (Lasix) IVP
  – 12-lead ECG = changes on anterior wall
• Underwent angioplasty; home within the week with good prognosis
	Mrs. Saunders is transported in an upright position on the cot with oxygen by nonrebreathing mask. An ALS unit provided IV, ECG monitoring, 3 doses of sublingual nitroglycerin, furosemide (Lasix) per protocol, and completed a 12-lead ECG which showed ST changes in V_3 and V_4, the anterior leads.
	
	Communication with the base physician allowed Mrs. Saunders to be met by the cardiac team who took her to the cardiac cath lab for angioplasty. Mrs. Saunders was sent home after one week.

Slide #25 **Case Study 3** • 72-year-old man, Mr. Brewer, complains of chest pain • Was raking leaves when pain started • M: Took 2 nitroglycerin before calling 9-1-1 • G: Pain feels like his last heart attack.	You are called to the home of a 72-year-old man, Mr. Brewer, who is complaining of substernal chest pain. He says that he was raking leaves when it started and he came in to rest and take his nitroglycerin. He took two tablets before he called 9-1-1 but got no relief (consider the "M" in the GEMS diamond). He is scared because the pain is just like his previous heart attack (consider the "G" in the GEMS diamond).

Section 2: Lectures

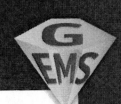

Slide Text	Additional Information
Slide #26 **Case Study 3 (continued)** • Mr. Brewer is pale, cool, and sweaty. • Pulse = 110 beats/min, respirations = 24 breaths/min, BP = 130/84 mm Hg • He states no relief from nitroglycerin. • He is nauseous, complains of SOB. *How can aging affect the body's interpretation of cardiac pain?* *How should you manage Mr. Brewer?*	Mr. Brewer is pale, cool, and clammy. He has a pulse of 110 beats/min, respirations of 24 breaths/min, and a blood pressure of 130/84 mm Hg. He has not received any relief from his nitroglycerin tablets. He is complaining of nausea and shortness of breath. *How can aging affect the body's interpretation of cardiac pain?* **(Elicit answers.)** *How should you manage Mr. Brewer?* **(Elicit answers.)** ***Discuss local management protocols.***
Slide #27 **Case Study 3 Conclusion** • Mr. Brewer received high-flow oxygen. • Nitroglycerin x 3 • Call made to cardiac team • Mr. Brewer taken to cath lab • Discharged home after one week • **ALS:** IV, monitor, 12-lead ECG, aspirin, morphine	Mr. Brewer received high-flow oxygen, and BLS assisted him with another dose of his nitroglycerin. ALS provided an IV, cardiac monitor, and 12-lead ECG which showed inferior wall ischemia. An additional 3 nitroglycerin were given as well as 324 mg of aspirin and 4 mg of morphine. The cardiac team was mobilized by the base physician. Shortly after arrival, Mr. Brewer was taken to the cardiac cath lab for angioplasty. He was discharged home after one week in the hospital.
Slide #28 **Summary** • Cardiac diseases are the number one cause of death. • COPD and pneumonia are 4th and 5th. • Respiratory and cardiac diseases are more likely in later years. • Older adults require thorough assessment, treatment, and transportation for respiratory and cardiac complaints.	Diseases of the heart are the number one cause of death in the older population. COPD and pneumonia are numbers 4 and 5, respectively. Due to age, the older body is more likely to acquire a respiratory or cardiac disease than a younger adult. Older adults require a thorough assessment to determine the needs for treatment and transportation. This may require sifting through a longer medical history than that of a younger adult.

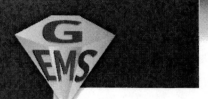

Section 2: Lectures

Elder Abuse and Neglect

Teaching Tips

The topic of elder abuse and neglect can be emotionally charged and discussing it may not be comfortable for all students. However, recognizing abuse and neglect and getting the patient on the way to appropriate treatment or services is critical.

A powerful way to start this lecture is to incorporate a story about an emergency call that involved potential abuse or neglect. For example, you could discuss why you thought there was potential abuse or neglect, what you did about it, and the outcome. Students could share stories of such calls as well.

Because local reporting requirements vary, this lecture requires slight customization. Find out your local reporting requirements prior to presenting this lecture. For example, if abuse or neglect is suspected, to whom should EMS report it, and in what form? Do certain documents need to be filled out? If possible, bring such a form and contact information to the class.

Also, it is a good idea to bring contact information for your state Ombudsman. The Ombudsman is responsible for ensuring that nursing homes adhere to laws regarding patient care and patient rights.

Providing contact information to students in the GEMS course will make them more likely to report suspected abuse or neglect than if you tell them to report it, but do not provide the means. Prepare as much relevant contact information as possible, for example in the form of a handout, before presenting the GEMS course. The handout could be distributed at the beginning of this lecture. Your efforts to prepare contact information will lead to better reporting and perhaps make the difference in getting an abused or neglected patient out of a bad situation.

Lecture Outline: Elder Abuse and Neglect

Slide Text	Additional Information
Slide #1 Elder Abuse and Neglect	This lecture covers topics found in Chapter 14: Elder Abuse and Neglect. *A powerful way to start this lecture is to incorporate a story about a personal experience you have had with elder abuse or neglect on an emergency call.*
Slide #2 **Objectives** • Define elder abuse. • Discuss who is at risk. • Describe the assessment of abuse. • Describe documentation of abuse.	*Read objectives.*

Section 2: Lectures

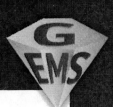

Slide Text	Additional Information
Slide #3 **Elder Abuse and Neglect** *What is elder abuse and neglect?* • Any form of mistreatment, or absence of care, that results in harm or loss to an older person • May include physical, sexual, or psychological abuse, or financial exploitation	*What is elder abuse and neglect?* Elder abuse is any form of mistreatment that results in harm or loss to an older person. This may include physical, sexual, or psychological abuse, or financial exploitation. An easy way to remember elder abuse is to think of it as inadequate care. Elder neglect is the absence of care. Examples of what results from neglect include urination or defecation in bed, pressure ulcers, poor nutrition, and nonadherence to medications.
Slide #4 **Profile of the Abused** • **S:** Older people at risk for abuse: – Women – Over 75 years – Live with abuser – Chronic physical or mental impairment – Socially isolated – Problematic behavior from the older person	Older people who are at risk of abuse fit a profile (consider the "S" in the GEMS diamond). These profiles can include: • Women • Over 75 years of age • Live with the abuser—this is commonly related to the amount of time that is required for care of the older person. • Chronic physical or mental impairment—physical conditions such as arthritis, COPD, cardiac problems, recent strokes or diabetes, and mental impairment as with Alzheimer's or other dementias can exceed the caregiver's ability to adequately care for the older person. • Socially isolated—those people who do not have social support are more easily abused, because no one may notice that abuse is occurring. Also, caregivers without adequate support from family, friends, or neighbors may become burned out and be more likely to abuse the patient. • Problematic behavior from the older person—incontinence, shouting out, constant calling for attention, or any action that requires the caregiver to stop and check on or care for the older person.

Section 2: Lectures

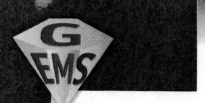

Slide Text	Additional Information
Slide #5 **Profile of an Abuser**<ul><li>Live with victim</li><li>Drug or alcohol users</li><li>Most over age 50</li><li>Dependent for financial support</li><li>Poor impulse control</li><li>History of domestic violence</li></ul>	Abusers also tend to fit a profile. Some of the common characteristics include:<ul><li>Live with victim—these persons usually care for the older person throughout the day and night.</li><li>Drug or alcohol users—abusers tend to have problems with drug or alcohol dependency.</li><li>Most are over 50 years of age.</li><li>Dependent for financial support—often the abuser cannot leave the older person because the older person is the abuser's only financial support. This may be through direct cash flow or they may own the house in which the abuser lives.</li><li>Poor impulse control</li><li>History of domestic violence—this can be against any other member of the household (eg, husband, child, brother, etc.).</li></ul>
Slide #6 **Patient Rights in Nursing Homes**<ul><li>Nursing Home Reform Amendments of OBRA 1987<ul><li>Right to self-determination</li><li>Personal and privacy rights</li><li>Rights regarding abuse and restraints</li><li>Rights to information</li><li>Rights to visits</li><li>Transfer and discharge rights</li></ul></li></ul>	The Nursing Home Reform Act as part of the Omnibus Reconciliation Act of 1987 (OBRA) introduced new requirements for quality of care, resident health assessment, care planning, use of medications, and physical restraints. The act mandates rights to the residents of these facilities. These rights include:<ul><li>Right to self-determination</li><li>Personal and privacy rights</li><li>Rights regarding abuse and restraints</li><li>Rights to information</li><li>Rights to visits</li><li>Transfer and discharge rights</li></ul>Refer to Table 14-1 in text.
Slide #7 **Ombudsman**<ul><li>One per state</li><li>Advocates for nursing home residents, relatives, and friends</li></ul>	The state Ombudsman can be a useful resource for EMS providers in cases of suspected abuse or neglect.

Section 2: Lectures

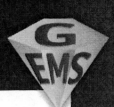

Slide Text	Additional Information
• Investigates quality of care, residents' complaints/concerns, and resolves them • Reports to licensing authority/law enforcement if abuse is suspected • Is a resource for EMS providers	The Long Term Care Ombudsman Program, authorized by the Older Americans Act, advocates for residents in nursing homes (and assisted living facilities in some states) and their relatives and friends. There is an Ombudsman in every state, territory, and the District of Columbia, usually housed in the state agency handling aging services (the State Unit on Aging). The responsibility of the Ombudsman is to be a presence in the facility, to receive and investigate quality of care and residents' rights complaints and concerns, and to resolve them if possible before crises occur. As with other health professionals, if the Ombudsman detects or suspects abuse, neglect or exploitation, a report is made to the licensing authority and law enforcement agencies.
Slide #8 **EMS Responsibilities** • Be a patient advocate. • Report suspected abuse/neglect to appropriate agency. • Document your assessment completely.	The responsibilities of EMS vary from state to state; however being a patient advocate is universal. Reporting requirements will also vary. (***Discuss the local requirements at this point.***) At a minimum, the suspected abuse should be reported to the ED staff receiving the patient. Documentation is important and is discussed later in this lecture.
Slide #9 **Red Flags** • Inadequate care • Poor environment • Patient fearful or hostile toward caregiver • Patient reluctant when questioned • Patient appears depressed • Conflicting accounts • Caregiver answers for patient • Lack of caregiver concern	There are several red flags for abuse and neglect. Keep the GEMS diamond in mind. Signs of inadequate care should be considered a red flag for potential abuse: • Abuse—poor hygiene, malnutrition, unmanaged medical problems, frequent falls, confusion • Neglect—poor hygiene, malnutrition, signs of deliberate self-injury

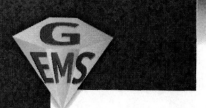

Section 2: Lectures

Slide Text	Additional Information
	A poor environment can be a sign of elder abuse or neglect. Check for: • Home in poor condition • Hazardous conditions (poor wiring, broken windows, clutter) • Temperature (too hot, too cold) • Fecal/urine odor • Presence of liquor bottles • Soiled bedding • Lack of smoke detectors • Patient confined • Expired/unmarked medications Interaction between the patient and caregiver can provide signals as to whether or not abuse or neglect is occurring. If the patient appears fearful of or hostile toward the caregiver or is reluctant to answer questions, or if the caregiver interrupts and answers for the patient, hovers around the patient, or prevents you from interacting with the patient, this may be a sign that the caregiver is an abuser. Conflicting accounts provided by the patient and caregiver can also signal abuse. If the patient appears depressed, this could be a sign of abuse or neglect. Investigate further and take measures to address potential depression or risk of suicide.
Slide #10 **Documentation** • Verbal and written reports • **E, S:** Include environmental and social assessments. • Include patient and caregiver quotes. • Document all injuries.	The patient care report will be the provider's ability to care for the elder abuse patient. Many people will read the report, including the ED staff, social services, law enforcement, and lawyers. Complete, accurate, and objective reports will ensure the future readers of your concerns. Your verbal report to the nurse and physician should include the same issues. Social interaction and environmental assessments are important because the EMS provider is the only person to see the patient in the home setting (consider the "E"

Section 2: Lectures

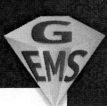

Slide Text	Additional Information
	and "S" in the GEMS diamond). None of the other professionals involved will be able to see what was seen at the time of the incident. Reports should include quotes from the patient or caregiver, especially when their stories do not agree. Injuries should be documented. Type of injury, location, multiple injuries, injuries of differing age, and injuries with patterns must be described clearly and objectively.
Slide #11 **Case Study 1** • Dispatched for 84-year-old Mrs. Brown with decreased LOC • S: Circumferential bruises of wrists, multi-colored bruising over lower back • Makes no eye contact with EMS	You are dispatched to the home of an 84-year-old woman, Mrs. Brown, for decreased level of consciousness. She is lying on the kitchen floor. Her eyes are open as you enter the room, but she makes no effort to acknowledge your arrival or respond to your questioning. During your assessment, you note circumferential bruises around both wrists and bruising over her lower back (consider the "S" in the GEMS diamond). Mrs. Brown's sister states that the patient sometimes becomes hard to handle, and that she fell last week and wouldn't accept help. Mrs. Brown immediately interrupts the conversation and states, "You pushed me." A verbal dispute ensues.
Slide #12 **Case Study 1 (continued)** • After careful assessment of the situation, you recommend transport to ED. • Mrs. Brown refuses treatment. *What are Mrs. Brown's rights?* *What can you do?*	In order to attempt to calm things down, you suggest getting Mrs. Brown evaluated in the ED. Mrs. Brown refuses treatment or transport. *What are Mrs. Brown's rights?* **(Elicit answers.)** Mrs. Brown is an adult and has the right to refuse care if she is competent. *What can you do?* **(Elicit answers.)** Talking to the patient and caregiver in a nonjudgmental way can take the EMS provider a long way. Showing genuine concern for the well-being of the patient can be a powerful tool.

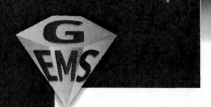

Section 2: Lectures

Slide Text	Additional Information
Slide #13 **Case Study 1 Conclusion** • Mrs. Brown refused services. • Police were contacted but were unable to charge sister with assault. • Brochures were left with Mrs. Brown for social services that were available in community.	Mrs. Brown continued to refuse treatment and transport to the ED. You were concerned for her welfare and contacted the police to come to the scene. Mrs. Brown refused to sign charges against her sister and the police had no other course of action. You received a signed refusal of services. Mrs. Brown was provided with brochures of services available in the community to help with the needs of the older population (food, housing, legal services).
Slide #14 **Case Study 2** • Dispatched to nursing home for 82-year-old Mr. Schmidt with altered mental status • Responsive to pain • E: Urine soaked, has new and old pressure ulcers	You are dispatched to the nursing home for altered mental status. The 82-year-old man, Mr. Schmidt, is lying in bed. Mr. Schmidt is responsive to painful stimuli only. However, your environmental exam shows a urine-soaked bed and Mr. Schmidt is wearing a diaper that doesn't appear to have been changed recently (consider the "E" in the GEMS diamond). He has pressure ulcers (bed sores) that appear red, inflamed, and open.
Slide #15 **Case Study 2 (continued)** • Vital signs and exam lead you to suspect sepsis. • Staff states Mr. Schmidt is difficult to care for. *Does the nursing home have the responsibility to care for the patient?* *Are there rules that define the patient's rights?*	Vital signs and assessment show a septic patient. When questioned, the staff member states that Mr. Schmidt is sometimes difficult and does not allow them to take care of him. *Does the nursing home have the responsibility to care for the patient?* **(Elicit answers.)** Yes. *Are there rules that define the patient's rights?* **(Elicit answers.)** Yes.
Slide #16 **Case Study 2 Conclusion** • Mr. Schmidt allowed transport after reassurance. • Suspicion of abuse was reported to ED.	After making the effort to talk to Mr. Schmidt, he stops fighting you and allows you to transport him to the hospital. You report the suspicion of abuse to the attending ED physician, who files a report with the appropriate agencies.

Section 2: Lectures

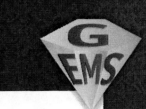

Slide Text	Additional Information
Slide #17 **Summary** • Elder abuse is mistreatment that results in harm. • Older people at risk include women and individuals over age 75. • Evaluation of abuse should include physical, social, and environmental assessments. • Careful documentation of abuse is needed for continued patient care.	*Review summary.*

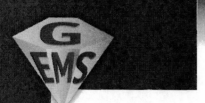

Section 2: Lectures

(ALS) Pharmacology and Medication Toxicity Emergencies

Teaching Tips

This lecture is specifically designed for the ALS GEMS course only, as ALS providers have more initial training in pharmacology and are able to administer some medications.

Throughout this lecture, it would be useful to mention the drug class when discussing certain types of drugs. Some newer providers may not be familiar with exact drugs, but will better understand what is being discussed if they understand the drug type and the effects it has on the body.

Prior to the course, consider calling several local pharmacies and inquiring about several prices of medications that the older patient may be taking. This information can be used during the discussion of nonadherence due to economic causes.

As in other lectures, tie-in material from Lecture 2: Changes with Age where applicable. This is relevant throughout much of the lecture, for example, when discussing drug absorption in an older person's body and how it can relate to polypharmacy.

Lecture Outline: Pharmacology and Medication Toxicity Emergencies

Slide Text	Additional Information
Slide #1 Pharmacology and Medication Toxicity Emergencies	This lecture covers topics found in Chapter 13: Pharmacology and Medication Toxicity Emergencies.
Slide #2 Objectives • Discuss physiological changes in older people with regard to the effects of medication on the body. • Describe the epidemiology of medication emergencies in the older population.	*Read objectives.*
Slide #3 Objectives (continued) • Discuss the assessment of medication toxicity and medication nonadherence. • Discuss the intervention, treatment, and transport of these patients. • Discuss ways EMS providers can help prevent medication misuse.	*Read objectives.*

Section 2: Lectures

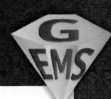

Slide Text	Additional Information

Slide #4
Passage of Drugs Through the Body
• Absorption
• Distribution
• Metabolism and elimination
  – Kidneys
  – Liver
	Absorption
	• There is some slowing of the digestive process secondary to decreased gastric acidity and slowed gastric emptying. This has little effect on speed of absorption of PO medications.
	
	Distribution
	• Lean body mass and reduction of body water and the increase in body fat alter the absorption of some medications. The lower water content results in higher blood concentrations of drug. Higher body fat allows for accumulation of fat-soluble drugs.
	
	Metabolism and elimination:
	• Kidneys—reduction in renal blood flow and the size and number of nephrons slow filtration and elimination of renal excreted drugs.
	• Liver—metabolism is slowed because of a reduction in liver mass, and decreased blood flow.

Slide #5 **Changes to the Therapeutic Effect of Drugs** • Drug interactions • Drug-drug interactions • Drug-nutrient interactions • Drug-disease interactions • Drug-herb interactions	Increased risk of adverse drug events is compounded in the older population by physiological changes effecting distribution, elimination, and drug interactions. Older patients are generally considered to have increased potency to medications. Drug interactions occur with multiple prescriptions, food, disease states, and drug toxicity. Increase in the number of drugs used, mixing of alcohol, and/or over-the-counter medications can precipitate reactions. Drug-drug interactions occur with alteration of the pharmacokinetics/pharmacodynamics of at least one of the medications (see Table 13-1 in textbook). Interactions can be potentiation, synergism, antagonism, or other harmful effects of drugs.

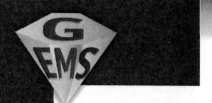

Section 2: Lectures

Slide Text	Additional Information
	Drug-nutrient interactions are predominantly caused by alteration of the absorption. Some medications can be effected directly by foods. Grapefruit juice can affect many classes of medications including: Versed, Mevacor, Zocor, some cyclosporin antibiotics, and prescription antihistamines such as Seldane.
	Drug-disease interactions are caused by one or more medications acting to worsen an existing disease. Sometimes atypical presentation manifests as confusion (see Table 13-2 in textbook). An example is the effect a non-steroidal anti-inflammatory can have on the kidney. This can lower the blood pressure or even place a patient at risk for developing CHF.
	Drug-herb interactions are not well documented, although it is felt that the occurrence is rare. However some common herbal remedies are becoming popular and obtaining a history of usage should be included. An example could include Ginkgo-biloba, which can increase the effects of an anti-coagulant.

Slide #6
Medication Assessment
• A comprehensive medication history is crucial.
• **M**: Barriers
   – Cognitive impairment
   – Underreporting
	In identifying drug-related problems, it is imperative to obtain a comprehensive medication history. The next slides will provide a map of how to assess an older person's medications.
	
	Barriers in the older patient can include cognitive impairment and underreporting (consider the "M" in the GEMS diamond). Cognitive barriers include forgetting what medications to take or when to take them. Underreporting occurs when a patient does not want to tell providers what medications he or she took.

Section 2: Lectures

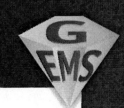

Slide Text	Additional Information
Slide #7 **Medication History** • Prescribed medications • Adherence • OTC medications • Herbal remedies • Other sources	Completing a medication history is an important part of the history of an older patient. Older people purchase as much as 25% of all prescribed medications and 33% of all over-the-counter medications sold in the U.S. The next slides will look at the components of the medication history.
Slide #8 **Prescribed Medications** • Get complete list, including doses. • Check prescribing doctor. • Look for new medications. • Ask about stopped medications.	When completing a medication history, list all of the medications that the patient is taking and their prescribed dosages. When copying the information from the medication containers, look for multiple prescribing physicians. Many patients have different physicians for different problems; this can be a reason for polypharmacy. Look for new medications or medications that have been recently stopped as these may be reasons for common complaints.

Slide #9
Adherence
• Prescriptions
  – Determine if medications are taken as prescribed.
  – Assess if medications are prescribed and not taken.
• OTC and herbal medications
  – List all that are taken.
  – Determine why they are taken.
	Question the patient to see if the medications are taken as prescribed. Do they understand the instructions? Can they read them? Are there any medications that the patient is supposed to be taking but is not? This may happen because the patient cannot afford them or does not like the side effects.
	
	Many over-the-counter (OTC) medications can interfere with prescribed medications. Some of these are well known—such as taking aspirin and warfarin (Coumadin)—others are not as obvious. List all of the OTC and herbal remedies that the patient is taking in your history. Also try to determine why the patient is taking the remedy. It may be to control a side effect of one of the prescribed medications.

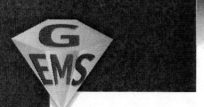

Section 2: Lectures

Slide Text	Additional Information

Slide #10
Other Sources
• Obtain thorough medication history.
  – Has patient taken another person's medications?
• E: Assess environment.
  – Is there evidence of alcohol or illicit drug usage?
	There are many sources of drugs that the older patient has access to. A spouse, sibling, or child's medication may seem like it will help the problem. You may find a patient saying, "It always works for my wife."
	
	Be astute during your environmental exam (consider the "E" in the GEMS diamond). Is there evidence of drug or alcohol usage? Alcohol is widely used in the older population and can affect other medications. An example is alcohol increasing the effects of a sedative such as alprazolam (Xanax).

Slide #11
Common Adverse Drug Events
• Cardiovascular
  – Dizziness, syncope, falls
• CNS
  – Confusion, psychiatric symptoms
• GI
  – Nausea, vomiting
	There are three main body systems affected by adverse drug events: cardiovascular, CNS, and the GI system. These events are often difficult to detect in older patients.
	
	Orthostatic hypotension is the most common adverse effect on the cardiovascular system (see Table 13-4 in textbook).
	
	The most common CNS effects are confusion and psychiatric symptoms (see Table 13-5 in textbook).
	
	Common GI problems are nausea, vomiting, and nutritional problems.

Slide # 12
Other Common Categories of Adverse Events
• Anticholinergic
  – Mental confusion
  – Dry eyes, mouth
  – Constipation, urinary retention
• Metabolic
  – Hypokalemia, hyponatremia, or low bicarbonate
	Over-the-counter antihistamines are the main causes of anticholinergic problems. Traditionally OTC antihistamines are the main problem.
	
	Diphenhydramine (Benadryl) can be found in cold and allergy products as well as Tylenol PM. These can cause confusion, dryness of the eyes and mouth, constipation, and urinary retention.
	
	Other common adverse drug reactions include hypokalemia, hyponatremia, and low bicarbonate. These metabolic disturbances can be caused by the medications themselves like when a diuretic also spills potassium. Hypoglycemia is also the result of a metabolic disturbance.

Section 2: Lectures

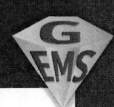

Slide Text	Additional Information

Slide #13
Drug Withdrawal Problems
• Adverse drug withdrawal event
  – Worsening of disease
  – Withdrawal reaction
• Reasons for nonadherence
	A patient's unilateral, intentional discontinuation of a drug can cause an adverse drug withdrawal event (ADWE).
	
	This can cause exacerbation of the underlying disease, and can occur months after cessation of the medication.
	
	Manifestation of the disease can worsen, or physiological withdrawal reaction (see Table 13-7 in textbook).
	
	Reasons for nonadherence can be to avoid side effects, feeling that they are fine without the medication, or economic.

Slide #14 **Nonadherence and Its Risks** • Increased morbidity/mortality • Increased healthcare costs • Increased hospital stays	An ever-increasing older population will result in increased nonadherence. Factors that contribute to this: • Forgetting to take medications on time • Not remembering the correct amount or dose • Poor technique with medication administration devices • Difficulty understanding label/directions • Difficulty opening containers • Financial problems (cannot afford medications)
Slide #15 **Intervention, Management, and Transport** • Event-dependent intervention is required. • Consider administration of antagonists. • Use caution in treatment.	Event-dependent intervention is required. In most overdoses, the most important treatment is maintaining ABCs. Consider administration of antagonists. Antagonists such as calcium for a calcium channel blocker, or naloxone (Narcan) for an opiate overdose can be lifesaving interventions. Use caution in treatment. Remember that small doses of medications may have been enough to put the patient over the edge. Quickly reversing some of these medications may be more dangerous than the current symptoms.

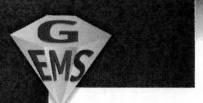

Section 2: Lectures

Slide Text	Additional Information
Slide #16 **Prevention of Medication Misuse** • Collect all medications, take to ED • Assess if patient is taking medications exactly as indicated. • Assess body systems with problems that may be due to side effects. • Encourage patients to carry complete, current medication list at all times.	As EMS providers, we are in a unique position to assist the older population with medication questions and concerns. We are invited into their homes and given access to their personal history. Collect all of the medications by bottle or by history and have the ED physician evaluate them all together. This may be the only time that a physician has seen all of the medications together. Assess the situation to determine if the patient understands the instructions for taking the medications. Try to correct them if possible or bring this to the attention of the attending staff when you arrive at the hospital. Many medications have side effects that are uncomfortable to the patient. Have the patient keep a list and discuss them with their doctor before they stop taking necessary medications. Encourage patients to make a list of their current medications and to carry it with them. This will not only make our job easier, but when they visit their doctor or pharmacist they will be able to discuss possible interactions.
Slide #17 **Case Study 1** • Dispatched to nursing facility for unresponsive 76-year-old Mr. Varne, prone in bed • Staff states he has been this way all morning. • Normally vocal and difficult to manage	Your service is dispatched to a nursing facility for an unconscious patient. Upon arrival you find a 76-year-old man, Mr. Varne, prone in bed, unresponsive. The staff states that he has been this way all morning. Mr. Varne normally is quite vocal and difficult to manage.
Slide #18 **Case Study 1 (continued)** • Pulse = 104 beats/min • Respirations = 28 breaths/min • BP = 124/84 mm Hg • Shallow respirations	Your examination reveals tachycardia with normal BP and shallow respirations, coupled with some peripheral tremors. Mr. Varne's record shows that the physician put him on the antipsychotic haloperidol (Haldol), 5 mg hs (hora somni, hour of sleep, at bedtime)

Section 2: Lectures

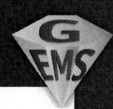

Slide Text	Additional Information
• Peripheral tremors • **M:** Record shows haloperidol (Haldol), 5 mg hs prescribed two days ago to assist staff in controlling him.	two days ago to assist staff in controlling him (consider the "M" in the GEMS diamond). Upon questioning, the staff state that Mr. Varne was very subdued yesterday and was less abusive.

Slide #19
Case Study 1 Conclusion
• Mr. Varne overdosed because:
  – Prescribed dosage was too high.
  – He could not eliminate normally.
• Transported to hospital for evaluation.
• Haldol dose was changed.
	The physician placed Mr. Varne on the maximum dose of medication, probably because of staff complaints of difficulty controlling him. After the second dose was given, combined with the first dose residual, Mr. Varne became overdosed.
	
	He was transported to the hospital for further evaluation. His medication dosage was adjusted to accommodate his aging body systems.

Slide #20 **Case Study 2** • Dispatched to a residence for an uncontrollable epistaxis • 68-year-old Mrs. Escalera found holding a blood-soaked towel	Upon arrival, you find an obese 68-year-old woman, Mrs. Escalera, sitting on the sofa with her head back, holding her nose with a blood-soaked towel.
Slide #21 **Case Study 2 (continued)** • Uncontrollable nasal bleeding • BP = 210/160 mm Hg • Pulse = 136 beats/min • Respirations = 24 breaths/min • Flushed skin • History of hypertension • **M:** Stopped medications because of cost	Assessment reveals a conscious, alert patient with unmanaged, bright red bleeding from both nostrils. Mrs. Escalera's face is flushed with petechial hemorrhages on the nose and cheeks. Vital signs are a blood pressure of 210/160 mm Hg, a heart rate of 136 beat/min and bounding pulses, and respirations of 24 breaths/min with effortless exchange. Mrs. Escalera is under treatment for hypertension, but has not seen her physician for some time. She is prescribed diazoxide (Hyperstat), furosemide (Lasix), and potassium chloride (KCl). After some coaxing, Mrs. Escalera relates that she could no longer afford the co-pay on the medications, and she felt really well, so she stopped taking them about two months ago (consider the "M" in the GEMS diamond).

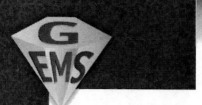

Section 2: Lectures

Slide Text	Additional Information
Slide #22 **Case Study 2 Conclusion** • Medication nonadherence for economic reasons • Medications were changed to generic brands. • Mrs. Escalera was enrolled in a prescription assistance program.	Mrs. Escalera stopped taking her medication, and the cumulative effect is the current hypertensive crisis. The hypertension has probably elevated gradually since she stopped taking her medication, but since hypertension is completely insidious, she was not aware of her worsening condition. Mrs. Escalera's medications were changed to generic prescriptions to assist her in maintaining adherence. She was also enrolled in a local prescription assistance program.
Slide #23 **Case Study 3** • Dispatched to residence of unresponsive 73-year-old • Mrs. Hart is lying supine on floor.	Upon arrival, you encounter a 73-year-old woman, Mrs. Hart, with her grandson in attendance. He states that he found her on the floor, unresponsive, when he arrived to check on her.
Slide #24 **Case Study 3 (continued)** • Pulse = 136 beats/min • Respirations = 28 breaths/min • BP = 180/94 mm Hg • Warm, dry skin • History of hypertension and diabetes • Meds: diazoxide (Hyperstat) and glyburide (Micronase) • **ALS:** Blood glucose reads HI	Assessment reveals a comatose patient lying on the floor with warm, dry skin. Vital signs are a blood pressure of 180/94 mm Hg, a heart rate of 136 beats/min with weak, thready pulses, and respirations of 28 breaths/min and deep (Kussmaul respirations). Mrs. Hart is under treatment for hypertension and type II diabetes. She is prescribed diazoxide (Hyperstat) and glyburide (Micronase). The grandson states that she has had increasing problems with mentation, and she has difficulty remembering to take, or if she has taken, her medications. **ALS:** A finger stick blood sugar test shows a blood glucose reading that is off the scale.

Section 2: Lectures

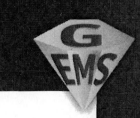

Slide Text	Additional Information
Slide #25 **Case Study 3 Conclusion** • You determine that Mrs. Hart's emergency is most likely hyperglycemia. • **ALS:** IV established and fluid bolus started • Mrs. Hart is transported for further evaluation and medication adjustment.	The grandson states that his grandmother does not like the way that the medication makes her feel and she often does not take it when she is feeling better. Mrs. Hart has had previous episodes of high blood pressure and hyperglycemia. **ALS:** IV therapy was initiated and a fluid bolus was started en route to the hospital. Mrs. Hart was admitted to the ICU and counseled regarding her usage of medications.
Slide #26 **Summary** • Aging changes how medications affect the body. • Older people experience problems with medications. • Assessment must include a comprehensive medication list. • Treatment may include use of antagonists. • EMS is in a unique position to help prevent medication misuse.	*Review slide.*

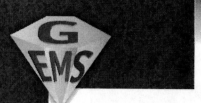

Section 2: Lectures

(ALS) Psychiatric Emergencies

Teaching Tips

EMS providers are not expected or trained to counsel older patients who are depressed or at risk for suicide. However, if the EMS provider does not notice signs of a psychiatric emergency or does not take steps to initiate treatment, a poor patient outcome or even death could result.

This lecture aims to teach students how to recognize a psychiatric emergency, or the potential thereof, in older patients. Depression, suicide, and substance abuse are discussed. Stress to students that the EMS provider may be the older person's only link to the health care system, and therefore, that investigating potential depression, suicidal intent, or alcohol abuse is an important part of every geriatric call. The "S" component of the GEMS diamond can be frequently integrated throughout this lecture.

This lecture provides another great chance to involve students and draw on their experiences with patients with psychiatric emergencies. Consider starting the lecture with a brief session asking students if they have encountered older patients who were depressed, suicidal, or potential abusers of alcohol. Throughout the lecture, provide tips that you may have from personal experience, and have students do the same.

Lecture Outline: Psychiatric Emergencies

Slide Text	Additional Information
Slide #1 **Psychiatric Emergencies**	This lecture covers topics found in Chapter 11: Psychiatric Emergencies. *Consider beginning the lecture by asking students if they have experienced emergency calls with older patients who were depressed, suicidal, or potential abusers of alcohol.*
Slide #2 **Objectives** • Describe the epidemiology of depression, suicide, and substance abuse in older people. • Identify the need for intervention and transport of the older patient experiencing a psychiatric emergency. • Develop a treatment plan for an older patient experiencing a psychiatric emergency.	*Read objectives.*

Section 2: Lectures

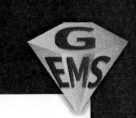

Slide Text	Additional Information
Slide #3 **Depression** • Common, debilitating psychiatric disorder • Affects 2 million older adults • 30% of older adults in nursing facilities suffer some form of clinical depression.	Depression is a common psychiatric disorder that is often debilitating. Depression is three times more likely to be diagnosed in women than men. Depression is different from the emotional experience of sadness or temporary "bad moods" because patient experiences it as extreme and persistent. Older people are at high risk for depression. As many as 2 million older adults may experience depression. 30% of older adults in skilled nursing facilities suffer some form of clinical depression. This population is the most likely to experience some form of depression.
Slide #4 **Red Flags for Depression** • Frequent non-urgent calls or ED/doctor visits • Severity of complaint unequal to findings • Personal neglect • Lack of social support • Loss of sense of enjoyment	Red flags for depression include: • Frequent non-urgent calls • Frequent ED or doctor visits • Severity of complaint unequal to findings • Personal neglect • Lack of social support • Loss of sense of enjoyment (anhedonia) Refer to the Geriatric Depression Scale (Table 11-1) to see how to assess an older person's level of depression.
Slide #5 **Management of Depression** • Patients suffering depression should be transported for evaluation. • Treatment usually includes medication or therapy. • S: Social networks can also help individuals fight depression.	Treatment of depression in the older adult consists of counseling and medications. The older patient with depression should be transported to a facility capable of diagnosing and treating the condition. The "S" (social) evaluation of the patient's social network can help in the treatment of depression. Individuals with an active social network are better able to fight depression.
Slide #6 **Suicide** • Older males have one of the highest rates.	Older people are at a high risk for suicide. Older males have one of the highest suicide rates of any age group. Older people experience many risk

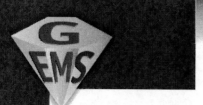

Section 2: Lectures

Slide Text	Additional Information
• Older people use more lethal means. • Men commit suicide 4 times more than women.	factors for depression and suicide as part of growing older. The death of a loved one, physical illness, isolation (or a smaller social network), and a loss of meaning in life all contribute to depression and suicidal thoughts. Older people use the most lethal means available to commit suicide. Because of this and their high level of risk, suicide is often successful and any hint a patient may want to commit suicide should be taken very seriously. Men commit suicide 4 times more often then women, but women attempt suicide 3 times more often. Men will often use firearms, while females tend to use less lethal methods.
Slide #7 **Circumstances that Increase Risk for Suicide** • Death of a loved one • Physical illness • Depression • Isolation • Substance abuse • Loss of life roles	Circumstances that increase risk for suicide include: • Death of a loved one, especially a life long partner • Physical illness—diseases that are chronic tend to wear the patient down over time • Depression—as mentioned earlier, this is a major problem in the older population • Isolation—loss of a social network limits the patient's ability to deal with depression • Substance abuse—this is a major cause for depression in all ages • Loss of life roles—changes in the person's position in life can lead to feelings of worthlessness. Retirement changes the older person's role in society. For example, a man who was the boss at work and the breadwinner at home is no longer either of those once he retires.
Slide #8 **Red Flags for Suicidal Patients** • Preoccupation with death • Giving away prized possessions • Taking unnecessary risks	Red flags for suicide include: • Preoccupation with death • Giving away prized possessions • Taking unnecessary risks • Increased use of alcohol/drugs

Section 2: Lectures

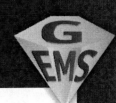

Slide Text	Additional Information
• Increased use of alcohol/drugs • Medication nonadherence • Getting a weapon	• Medication nonadherence • Acquiring a weapon Pay special attention to these signs. They may be subtle, and you may be the patient's best chance at diagnosis and treatment before he or she commits suicide.
Slide #9 **Management of a Suicidal Patient** • Ask if patient is contemplating suicide. • Take patient seriously. • Secure dangerous items. • Transport potentially suicidal patients. • Report concerns to ED. • Do not leave patient unattended. • Offer hope.	If you suspect an older patient to be depressed or suicidal: • Take patient seriously. • Ask if patient is contemplating suicide. • Secure dangerous items. • Transport potentially suicidal patients. • Report concerns to ED. • Do not leave patient unattended (unless required to in order to achieve scene safety). • Offer hope.
Slide #10 **Substance Abuse** • Includes misuse and abuse of alcohol, illicit drugs, and medications • Underdetected in older population, but about 10% are chemically dependent • Variety of medications for chronic conditions increases likelihood of medication problems	Substance abuse includes abuse and misuse of alcohol and medications, both prescription and over the counter. Substance abuse in the older population is largely underdetected and undiagnosed. This may be because family members are ashamed or embarrassed, or because the older adult is not in criminal difficulties with police, not violent, and less likely to be involved in a DUI motor vehicle crash. Also, many older people live alone and lack some type of support system, making it less likely that substance abuse will be detected or diagnosed. *(At this point, ask students to brainstorm for reasons why an older person might abuse or misuse a substance.)* Reasons for increased alcohol and medication abuse can include going from a productive career to an unexpected, unwanted retirement, loss of a spouse, or boredom.

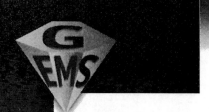

Section 2: Lectures

Slide Text	Additional Information
Slide #11 **Misuse** • Older people make up an eighth of the population, but use a third of prescription medications. • Misuse can be: – Intentional (suicide attempt) – Unintentional (trouble reading label)	Older people make up about one eighth of the population, but use almost one third of prescription medications. Because of the many medications they are on, older people are more likely to have medication problems such as medication interactions. Medication misuse can be intentional or unintentional. Older people may have trouble reading prescription directions due to visual impairments, or may be embarrassed to ask their doctor to clarify the instructions. Older people may intentionally misuse medications to inflict self-harm or commit suicide.
Slide #12 **Management of Substance Abuse** • Provide a complete medication history. • Provide contact info for social service agencies and crisis hotlines. • Consider making initial contact for patient.	If you suspect substance abuse in an older patient, review all medication regimens carefully. Ask about both prescription and over-the-counter medications. Provide contact information for social service agencies or crisis hotlines in your community. Consider making the initial call on behalf of the patient. Some patients will let you help them by making the first call. Check when and where an AA meeting will be taking place, or call a crisis line and initiate the beginning of the conversation. These may be a big help for the patient who wants help but is afraid to ask for it. Refer to Appendix A and www.GEMSsite.com for organizations and services for older people.
Slide #13 **Case Study 1** • Dispatched to an older patient with an overdose • 86-year-old Mr. Davis reportedly took a bottle of Xanax. • Mr. Davis is sleepy and refuses to answer questions.	You are dispatched to an overdose. An 86 year-old man, Mr. Davis, reportedly took a bottle of alprazolam (Xanax), an anti-anxiety drug and depressant. He appears sleepy but answers all of your questions appropriately.

Section 2: Lectures

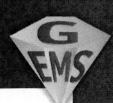

Slide Text	Additional Information
Slide #14 **Case Study 1 (continued)** • **S:** Per friend, Mr. Davis said he was "going to end it all." • **S:** Depressed since wife died • Pulse = 88 beats/min • Respirations = 12 breaths/min, • BP = 126/84 mm Hg • Pulse Ox = 96% • No trauma noted on exam • **S:** Empty bottle found	During your assessment, the patient's friend appears and states that Mr. Davis called and told him he was "going to end it all." He told him that he had a bottle of the depressants that he usually used to sleep and was going to take them all. The patient reports that he just doesn't have the will to go on since his wife died several months go (consider the "S" in the GEMS diamond). Your exam shows an older man who appears sleepy, with a pulse of 88 beats/min, respirations of 12 breaths/min, a blood pressure of 126/84 mm Hg, a pulse Ox of 96% on room air, and normal sinus rhythm on the monitor. You note no trauma during your assessment, but find an empty bottle of alprazolam (Xanax), which the patient says he used up for sleeping. A count of the pills and check of the date reveals more pills are missing than can be accounted for.
Slide #15 **Case Study 1 (continued)** *Should Mr. Davis' possible suicide attempt be taken seriously?* *What should be done to treat him?*	*Should Mr. Davis' possible suicide attempt be taken seriously?* **(Elicit answers.)** Yes. *What should be done to treat him?* **(Elicit answers.)** Treatment may include involving the police, social services, or other agencies depending on your local protocols. The possibility of suicide in this patient is real and he should receive additional medical care.
Slide #16 **Case Study 1 Conclusion** • Mr. Davis was taken into custody by police and admitted to hospital. • Admitted to taking Xanax to try to kill himself • Was enrolled in outpatient therapy after leaving hospital	The police were called and talked with Mr. Davis, whose speech was becoming slurred and was having a hard time staying awake. The police took him into protective custody. He was released to EMS for transport to the hospital. There he admitted to taking the pills in an attempt to kill himself. Mr. Davis was enrolled in outpatient therapy after a short stay in the hospital.

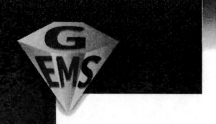

Section 2: Lectures

Slide Text	Additional Information
Slide #17 **Case Study 2** • Dispatched to intoxicated 66-year-old Mrs. Jones who fell outside liquor store • Has slurred speech, laceration over her eye, cannot get up off sidewalk	You are called to an intoxicated patient. 66 year-old Mrs. Jones fell on her way into the local liquor store this afternoon. She has slurred speech, a laceration over her left eye (with minor bleeding), and cannot seem to get up off the sidewalk. She has the smell of alcohol on her breath and states that she has been drinking.
Slide #18 **Case Study 2 (continued)** • Pulse = 96 beats/min • Respirations = 22 breaths/min • Blood pressure = 190/100 mm Hg • Pulse Ox = 97% • **ALS:** ECG = NSR • $\frac{1}{2}$" laceration over left eye, bleeding has stopped • **M:** States she does not take her BP medication because she cannot have it with alcohol	Her pulse is 96 beats/min, respirations of 22 breaths/min, a blood pressure of 190/100 mm Hg, pulse Ox of 97% on room air, her ECG is normal sinus rhythm, and her blood sugar is 102 mg/dL. She has a $\frac{1}{2}$" laceration over her left eye with bleeding that has now stopped. She states she does not take her medication because her doctor told her not to mix it with alcohol (consider the "M" in the GEMS diamond).
Slide #19 **Case Study 2 (continued)** *What could have contributed to Mrs. Jones' fall?* *Should Mrs. Jones be allowed to RMA so she can go home and sleep it off?*	*What could have contributed to Mrs. Jones' fall?* **(Elicit answers.)** Syncope, trip on sidewalk, cardiac arrhythmia, medication misuse *Should Mrs. Jones be allowed to RMA so she can go home and sleep it off?* **(Elicit answers.)** The effects of alcohol can mask or alter the patient's assessment and your triage decision. This patient should be evaluated in the ED for additional injury or medical problems.

Section 2: Lectures

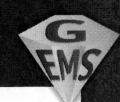

Slide Text	Additional Information
Slide #20 **Case Study 2 Conclusion** • Mrs. Jones was transported and evaluated at the ED. • Diagnosed with blood alcohol of 240 mg/dL and a subdural bleed • Sent to a nursing home for several weeks and then returned home	Mrs. Jones was transported to the local ED. She was diagnosed with a blood alcohol of 240 mg/dL (the equivalent of blowing 0.24 on a breathalizer test). She was, however, also diagnosed with a subdural bleed. Subdural bleeds are hard to diagnose in the field due to the brain atrophy from aging and the alcoholism. She spent several weeks in a nursing home and was discharged home with follow up care.
Slide #21 **Summary** • Depression, suicide, and substance abuse occur in older people. • Treatment and transport of the older patient experiencing a psychiatric emergency requires safety first. • Psychiatric emergencies in older patients require evaluation by qualified personnel.	While psychiatric problems are not a normal part of aging, depression, suicide, and substance abuse are issues that exist in the older population. Treatment of a patient with a psychiatric emergency begins with safety first. The suicidal patient can be so intent on doing something that he or she may lash out at the EMS provider. Psychiatric emergencies require evaluation by qualified personnel. This may not be available at all emergency departments. Use your local protocol in choosing your destination.

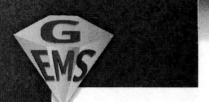

Section 2: Lectures

(Optional) Other Medical Emergencies

Teaching Tips

This lecture is optional and can be presented if you wish to provide a longer and more comprehensive GEMS course.

When presenting this lecture, as with others, try to incorporate stories from your personal experience regarding cases related to the topics discussed here. Particularly helpful would be a case in which it was difficult to identify the cause of the problem due to complexities such as previously existing conditions and multiple medications.

Lecture Outline: Other Medical Emergencies

Slide Text	Additional Information
Slide #1 **Other Medical Emergencies**	This lecture covers topics found in Chapter 12: Other Medical Emergencies.

Slide #2
Objectives
• Discuss the epidemiology and emergency care of the following emergencies in older patients:
  – Gastrointestinal
  – Malnutrition/dehydration
  – Endocrine
  – Integumentary
  – Sepsis
  – Environmental
	Read objectives.

Slide #3
GI Bleeding
• Upper GI bleeding
  – Esophagus to duodenum
  – NSAIDs
  – Alcohol
  – Esophageal varices, tears
• Lower GI bleeding
  – Typically colorectal
	Potential GI emergencies include:
	• Bleeding
	• Peptic ulcer disease
	• Obstruction
	• Nausea, vomiting, diarrhea
	• Constipation
	
	While the gastrointestinal system does not induce robust, acute life-threatening distress like the cardiac or respiratory systems, there can be conditions that have the potential to create medical emergency situations. Life-threatening hemorrhage

Section 2: Lectures

Slide Text	Additional Information
	or infection can result from urgent GI problems. Other GI conditions can require immediate surgical attention and involve EMS providers in the patient's stabilization and transfer.
	Upper GI bleeding typically occurs above the duodenum. Minor bleeding is typified by coffee ground emesis, whereas heavier bleeding presents as frank hematemesis and melena.
	Several risk factors are particularly noteworthy in older patients. Heavy NSAID use, for example in patients being treated for arthritis, may weaken the normal gastric protection mechanisms, leading to erosion of the stomach lining and bleeding.
	Chronic alcohol use/abuse can lead to gastric erosion and an increased risk of esophageal varices—each of which can present with significant bleeding that EMS providers cannot easily control. Older patients taking anticoagulants can even develop clinically significant residual bleeding from small esophageal tears after forceful vomiting.
	In marked contrast, lower GI bleeding presents rectally regardless of its origin. Keep in mind not to simply dismiss this bleeding as hemorrhoidal as the causes can be varied and the total amount of bleeding hidden.

Slide #4
Peptic Ulcer Disease
• Ulcers more likely with age
• NSAID use
• Dyspepsia/epigastric discomfort
• Bowel perforation
  – Fever
  – Abdominal rigidity
  – Silent abdomen
  – True surgical emergency
	Older patients are more likely to have gastric ulcers. Their stomachs have greater opportunities for erosion. This erosion can be accelerated by the factors mentioned in the previous slide for upper GI bleeding. Given the prevalence of chronic pain and altered perceptions of pain in the older population, the upper abdominal or epigastric burning of dyspepsia needs to be weighed carefully against your index of suspicion for cardiac chest discomfort.
	
	Erosions that lead to bowel perforation are true surgical emergencies. Gastric or intestinal contents in the abdomen can be devastating to the older patient.

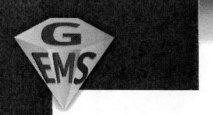

Section 2: Lectures

Slide Text	Additional Information
	Be alert for fever and abdominal pain. Be especially attuned to peritoneal signs of rigidity and a quiet bowel, as the symptoms and discomfort may be subtler in older patients.
Slide #5 **Intestinal Obstruction** • Adhesions • Volvulus • Masses • Nausea, vomiting • Dehydration	Bowel obstructions may be the cause of unexplained nausea and vomiting. These obstructions can occur from the adhesions from surgery, the bowel knotted upon itself (volvulus), or tumors inside the intestine or compressing it from the surrounding abdomen. The vomiting usually appears abruptly and may have a yellow-green character to it. Persistent vomiting, lack of intake, and intestinal absorption may result in dehydration.
Slide #6 **Nausea, Vomiting, Diarrhea** • 1,000 older people die from diarrheal illness • Dehydration • Electrolyte abnormalities • Incontinence	The symptom of nausea and signs of vomiting and diarrhea have poor specificity, so you need to be aware of the potential causes and consequences. Diarrheal illnesses can be fatal, especially among those institutionalized and being artificially fed. EMS providers should seek additional historical clues, characteristics (blood, color, etc.), and chronology for these signs and symptoms. Good history taking is essential to accurate diagnosis by the rest of the health care team. Nausea inhibits intake and vomiting and diarrhea induce losses of fluids, electrolytes, and nutrients. Diarrhea is not always reported by the older patient because of embarrassment. Such "accidents" should be recognized as largely involuntary and the patient's cleanliness and dignity addressed.
Slide #7 **Diverticulitis** • Sac-like bubbles • Infection prone • LLQ pain • Fistulas	Diverticula are pouch-like protrusions on the bowel that can become inflamed and infected, creating fever and abdominal pain. The abdominal pain is usually in the lower left quadrant, but can occur on the right side. The dangers of this condition are if connections are formed with other structures (fistulas) or perforations occur, allowing fecal matter to spread infection elsewhere in the abdomen.

Section 2: Lectures

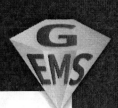

Slide Text	Additional Information

Slide #8
Gallbladder Disease
• Biliary colic
  – Sharp URQ pain, tenderness
• Gallstones
• Cholecystitis
  – Septic?
	Almost one-third of older patients have gallstones. Patients who wait for the symptoms to become severe have a poorer outcome from surgery. The discomfort of biliary colic is typically sharp upper right quadrant pain with tenderness that may change with deep extremes of breathing. Patients with this presentation may have infection (cholecystitis) if they are febrile and jaundiced. Your index of suspicion for sepsis should be heightened in these patients.

Slide #9
Elimination Disorders
• S: Incontinence
  – Impact on quality of life
  – Avoidance, social isolation
• Constipation
  – Fecal impaction
  – Prevention measures
    • Exercise
    • Fiber
    • Hydration
	Fecal incontinence is a reality in the older population. Because of the depression, embarrassment, and inconvenience associated with this problem, patients may avoid social situations. This can negatively affect their quality of life (consider the "S" in the GEMS diamond). Acute incontinence should be taken seriously as they may signal neurogenic complications of spinal injury or malignancy.
	
	Constipation is formally defined as less than one bowel movement every three days and is more common than fecal incontinence. Nearly one-third of older people deal with it, and may be too shy to reveal this to healthcare personnel. GI workup at the hospital is often effective. Patients who are institutionalized, sedentary, or those with Parkinson's disease may become constipated for more serious reasons such as fecal impaction. In this situation, hardened feces plug the sigmoid colon or rectum. Most constipation can be prevented by increasing activity, consuming an adequate amount of fiber-rich foods, or taking supplements with plenty of fluids.

Slide #10
Malnutrition and Dehydration
• Age-related factors
• E: Malnutrition:
  – Poorly nourished vs. undernourished
  – Chronic disease
  – S: Consider self-neglect.
	Malnutrition and dehydration are frequently coupled in the older population. Over time, total body water decreases because of declining muscle mass. A lack of activity encourages this loss of muscle and water. Declines in older patients' ability to smell, taste, and sense temperature act to diminish their motivation to eat or drink. Renal impairment

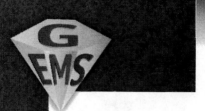

Section 2: Lectures

Slide Text	Additional Information

• Dehydration:
  – Dry mucous membranes.
  – Tachycardia
  – Poor urine output
	interferes with the body's ability to retain vital water reserves.
	
	Malnutrition in a general sense refers to patients who are poorly nourished. Obesity is the most common form of malnutrition. What is more commonly perceived as malnutrition is really undernourishment where there is an insufficient supply of nutrients for the body. This is typified by the thin, cachectic (emaciated) patient with loose clothing. You may note a lack of food in the home during your environmental assessment (consider "E" and "S" in the GEMS diamond).
	
	Detecting dehydration can be subtle. The key is not to rely on one finding, but collect several pieces to put the clinical picture together. Be attentive to the patient's weight, skin turgor, condition of mucous membranes, deviations in vital signs, flat neck veins, and poor urine output. Be aware that the patient's medications may mask these findings (beta blockers) or contribute to them (diuretics).

Slide #11
Endocrine Conditions
  • Interrelated with other body functions
  • Diabetes mellitus
  • Thyroid disorders
	Remember that the endocrine system is similar to the nervous system in that it is tightly interrelated to almost all body functions. While the types of endocrine abnormalities are many, the number that affect older patients and are of routine concern to EMS workers are few.
	
	Diabetes mellitus is by far the most common, affecting nearly one-fifth of the U.S. population. While diabetic emergencies in older patients are the same as in younger adults, older patients deal far more with the long-term complications of the disease such as acceleration of cardiovascular disease and kidney failure. Many patients discover they are diabetic after they have suffered a hyperglycemic complication.

Section 2: Lectures

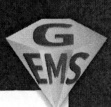

Slide Text	Additional Information

Slide #12
Hypoglycemia
 	
• Low blood sugar
• Rapid onset
• Easily reversed
• History of incident
   – Excessive demand/insulin
   – Insufficient carbohydrate intake
• **M:** Interfering medications
	Review these generally common characteristics with the audience.
	Remember that older patients taking beta blockers may not feel shaky or have the increased heart rate you would expect with low blood sugar. Also consider the "M" in the GEMS diamond.

Slide #13
Hyperglycemic Conditions
 	
• Diabetic ketoacidosis (DKA)
   – Lack of insulin
   – Body utilizes fat for energy
   – Byproducts are ketones and acids
• Nonketotic hyperglycemic-hyperosmolar coma (NKHHC)
   – Type II/NIDDM patients
   – Concurrent with abnormal demand
	The two hyperglycemic emergencies are no different in older patients.
	
	DKA results from a lack of insulin, forcing the body to look to fat for energy instead of carbohydrates. This alternative method produces ketones (that can be smelled in exhalation) and acids (which create Kussmaul respirations) in the extreme. Blood glucose levels of 300–500 mg/dL are not unusual in this condition. Treatment involves attention to the ABCs and oral glucose per local protocol. ALS providers will still monitor the blood glucose and provide IV fluids and insulin per medical control or local protocol.
	
	NKHHC is more commonly seen in older diabetics and must be aggressively treated because of its significant mortality. Blood glucose levels soar above 500 mg/dL and resulting neurologic problems such as seizures and coma can result. Situations of abnormal metabolic stress such as infection, trauma, and recovery after major surgery can trigger this emergency condition. Field treatment is similar to DKA.

Slide #14 **Thyroid Disorders** • Hypothyroidism – Cold, constipation, thinning hair, weight gain	The thyroid gland changes with age. Hypothyroidism prevalence rises with age and is more common in women and the institutionalized. The signs and symptoms are not very specific, so they are often dismissed to other causes.

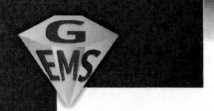

Section 2: Lectures

Slide Text	Additional Information

• Hyperthyroidism
  – Less spontaneous, more medication-induced
  – Hot, restlessness, tachycardia, palpitations, weight loss
• Thyroid storm
  – Fever, severe tachycardia, nausea/vomiting, CHF
	Hyperthyroidism occurs more from overmedication for hypothyroidism than on its own. It does not occur more frequently in older people, and affects genders equally. Feeling hot, agitated, and restless is typical in most adults but older patients have a larger proportion of cardiac findings such as CHF, chest pain, and atrial fibrillation.
	
	A severe version of hyperthyroidism is thyroid storm. These patients may become suddenly febrile, hyperdynamic (CHF, rapid atrial fibrillation), and nauseated with vomiting. Field treatment for these patients is largely supportive and includes arrhythmia management.

Slide #15
Integumentary Conditions
• Pressure ulcers
  – Decubitus ulcer, pressure sore, bedsore
  – Largely caused by healthcare process
  – Over bony prominences
  – Clinical stages
• Skin infections
	Though rarely true emergencies, the skin is the body's largest organ and does participate in various physiologic processes. Hence, attention to the skin in patients who may otherwise be medically frail is important.
	
	Many EMS tasks can create pressure ulcers. For example, repeated BP measurements in the same spot, prolonged immobilization to a backboard, and failure to change the older patient's position during lengthy transports all have the potential to create such sores. The majority of such ulcers occur in patients in medical facilities. The areas of greatest risk are those over bony areas of the body where the skin is easily compressed in a small area. Figure 12-20 in the text shows areas particularly vulnerable to pressure ulcer formation. Table 12-3 provides the scale used to grade the clinical stages of these wounds.
	
	During physical examination of older patients, be sure to document and respect areas of the skin with potential infection or inflammation. All rashes, ulcers, and discolorations that you note should be protected, recorded, and related to the receiving health care providers. Be sure to observe good infection control measures, including hand washing while caring for patients with potential skin infections.

Section 2: Lectures

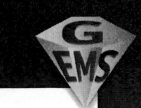

Slide Text	Additional Information

Slide #16
Infection and Sepsis
• Sepsis
• Bacteremia
• Septic shock
• Risk factors
  – Age-related
  – Institutionalization
	Infections are either bacterial, viral, or fungal. Sepsis is the syndrome that results from the effects of toxic products of these microorganisms in the bloodstream. It almost makes the Top Ten list of common causes of death in the U.S. Older patients have a harder time dealing with sepsis and it is frequently fatal. For this reason, providers need to sustain a high index of suspicion for sepsis. Febrile older patients who are both tachycardic and tachypneic are strong candidates for a sepsis work-up. When live organisms are abundant in the blood stream, this is referred to as septicemia. For example, if the organism is a bacterium, the patient is diagnosed with bacteremia.
	
	Septic shock results when there is compromised perfusion, hypotension, and/or respiratory status in a patient with sepsis.
	
	Age-related declines in immune function place older people at greater risk of sepsis than younger adults. Conditions such as malnutrition, cardiovascular disease, chronic pulmonary disease, and cancer all further predispose older people to infections and sepsis. Those already sick enough to have indwelling catheters and/or be institutionalized have greater opportunity to be infected by antibiotic-resistant organisms and spread that infection to other residents.

Slide #17
Sepsis
• Causes of sepsis
• Prevention
  – High index of suspicion
  – Universal precautions
  – Sterile technique for invasive care
  – Hand washing
	Sepsis can originate from infection in any body system. For example, pneumonia is the leading cause of death from infection in Americans older than 65. As already discussed, GI perforation, indwelling urinary catheters, and skin ulcers can be sources of infection.
	
	While treatment is largely supportive until the patient can receive prompt antibiotic treatment, prevention goes a long way in reducing overall morbidity and mortality. Universal precautions are essential. Respiratory care should employ meticulous sterile technique where appropriate. In fact, an oxygen mask on the patient's face serves a protective function for both provider and patient when needed.

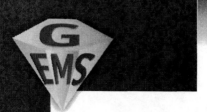

Section 2: Lectures

Slide Text	Additional Information
	Remember that hand washing is the single most important method to prevent the spread of infection in the health care setting. EMS providers should also stay up to date with all appropriate immunizations, including an annual flu shot.

Slide #18
Environmental Emergencies
• Thermoregulatory
   – Heat production
   – Heat loss
• Hypothermia
• Hyperthermia
• Prevention
	The most common environmental emergencies in older patients include heat disorders and hypothermia. The body's main "thermostat" is the hypothalamus at the base of the brain. It works with thermoreceptors throughout the body to regulate temperature. The body produces heat by various metabolic processes and shivering if necessary. Cooling happens from heat losses via the skin and respiratory systems. Thermoregulatory impairment makes older people more susceptible to hot/cold environmental emergencies. Those on fixed incomes may not be able to afford to set the temperature to comfortable level in their homes.
	
	Hypothermia is of larger concern in the older population. Hypothermia victims older than age 75 are five times more likely to die than younger counterparts. Thinner skin provides less insulation and more heat loss. Decreased muscle mass reduces the effectiveness of shivering. Chronic conditions and medications can also interfere with this thermoregulatory process. The treatment approach for older hypothermia victims is no different than other adults.
	
	Risk for hyperthermic heat emergencies is worsened by chronic medical conditions. The traditional syndromes of heat cramps, exhaustion, and stroke often present more severely in the older population. 80% of heat stroke deaths occur in people over 50 years old. Many medicines influence the body's ability to deal with heat stress. However, the treatment approaches for these hyperthermic conditions is no different than other adults, as well. EMS providers can help with efforts to monitor older people in the hot and cold seasons as one means of prevention.

Section 2: Lectures

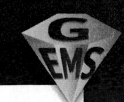

Slide Text	Additional Information
Slide #19 **Case Study 1** • Dispatched to 70-year-old Mr. Morgan • Normally exercises, but recently inactive since leg injury • Complains of persistent nausea, fatigue, tarry stool	You are dispatched to Mr. Morgan, a 70-year-old retired iron worker, for a complaint of persistent nausea, fatigue, and tarry stools. When you arrive at the scene, Mr. Morgan states that he normally exercises, but recently has been inactive because of a leg injury.
Slide #20 **Case Study 1 (continued)** • G: Arthritis, hypertension, MI • M: Ibuprofen, atenolol, aspirin • Physical exam: Pale skin • Respirations = 24 breaths/min; pulse = 88 breaths/min; BP = 110/90 mm Hg • Clear breath sounds, no JVD or edema *What is Mr. Morgan's likely problem?* *What factors confound your decision?*	*What is Mr. Morgan's likely problem?* **(Elicit answers.)** Your index of suspicion should be high for upper GI bleeding secondary to NSAID use and aggravated by routine aspirin use. Peptic ulcer disease with progressive anemia is another consideration, but the pallor and melena strongly point to bleeding. *What factors confound your decision?* **(Elicit answers.)** The beta blocker's ability to inhibit compensatory tachycardia may also confound attempts to estimate the severity of any blood loss.
Slide #21 **Case Study 1 Conclusion** • Mr. Morgan transported in position of comfort with high-flow oxygen by mask • History reveals recent increase in ibuprofen for new leg injury pain • Gastric bleeding identified by endoscopy and controlled • NSAID changed to allow stomach and leg to heal more comfortably	Mr. Morgan was transported in a position of comfort with high-flow oxygen by mask. The medication history revealed a recent increase in his ibuprofen intake to help with his leg injury pain. At the hospital, gastric bleeding was identified by endoscopy and was then controlled. Mr. Morgan's NSAID medication was changed to allow both his stomach and his leg to heal more comfortably.

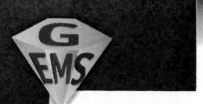

Section 2: Lectures

Slide Text	Additional Information
Slide #22 **Case Study 2** • Dispatched to nursing home for 82-year-old Miss Spring with AMS • Staff noticed she hasn't eaten well for past few days. • **G:** Non-insulin-dependent diabetes for 22 years	You are dispatched to a nursing home for an 82-year-old woman named Miss Spring. The nursing home staff called EMS because Miss Spring has altered mental status. When you arrive, the staff tells you that Miss Spring has not eaten well for the past few days. Also, Miss Spring has had non-insulin-dependent diabetes for the past 22 years (consider the "G" in the GEMS diamond). *Solicit early clinical impressions from the audience.*
Slide #23 **Case Study 2 (continued)** • **G:** NIDDM, arrhythmia • **M:** Glyburide, digoxin, multivitamin • Physical exam: Rambling, confused, slightly cool skin peripherally • Respirations = 16 breaths/min, pulse = 56 beats/min, BP = 108/58 mm Hg • **ALS:** Blood glucose = 102 mg/dL, ECG = slow atrial fibrillation *What is your opinion of Miss Spring's problem?*	You note that patient has a history of arrhythmia, takes digoxin, and shows atrial fibrillation. This was probably pre-existing (consider the "G" and "M" in the GEMS diamond). The physical exam reveals that the patient rambles and is confused. Her skin is slightly cool peripherally. Her respirations are 16 breaths/min, pulse is 56 beats/min, and her blood pressure is 108/58 mm Hg. The nursing staff states the patient has been compliant with all her medications. **ALS:** Her blood glucose is 102 mg/dL and the ECG shows slow atrial fibrillation. *What is your opinion of Miss Spring's problem? (Elicit answers.)*
Slide #24 **Case Study 2 Conclusion** • Miss Spring transported with oxygen, ECG monitoring • **ALS:** IV normal saline KVO • Hypothyroidism successfully treated by medication.	Miss Spring's decreased appetite (and therefore decreased intake) and confusion is offset by the fact that her blood glucose is near normal. This helps rule out the most common suspicions of hypoglycemia or diabetic emergency. It is worthwhile to recall that the prevalence of hypothyroidism rises with age, is higher in women, and is higher in institutionalized older patients. The bradycardia is a helpful observation here, as the heart rate would otherwise be rapid, reflecting the sympathetic response to hypoglycemia.

Section 2: Lectures

Slide Text	Additional Information
	Miss Spring was transported with oxygen and ECG monitoring. **ALS:** ALS administered IV normal saline at a keep-the-vein-open rate. Miss Spring was determined to have hypothyroidism and was successfully treated with medication.
Slide #25 **Case Study 3** • Dispatched to 78-year-old Mrs. Perkins • Has Alzheimer's, lives in a gated ward • Nursing staff ask for patient transport to hospital for fever, dark urine in recently-placed Foley catheter	You are dispatched to a 78-year-old woman, Mrs. Perkins, who is a retired office manager. She has Alzheimer's disease and lives in a gated ward. Upon arrival, the nursing staff asks you to transport the patient to the hospital due to her fever and dark urine draining in a recently-placed Foley catheter.
Slide #26 **Case Study 3 (continued)** • **G:** Alzheimer's, COPD, urinary incontinence • **M:** Aricept, Singulair, Flovent • Physical exam: Frequent congested cough; warm, flushed skin • Respirations = 28 breaths/min, pulse = 100 beats/min, BP = 100/60 mm Hg • No JVD or edema, but has crackles, rhonchi; deep orange urine in Foley bag *What is your impression of the problem?*	Note that mental status changes will be harder to assess because of the baseline dementia. Mrs. Perkins' history reveals Alzheimer's disease, COPD, and urinary incontinence. Her medications include Aricept, Singulair, and Flovent (consider the "G" and "M" in the GEMS diamond). The physical exam reveals a frequent, congested cough, and warm, flushed skin. Her respirations are 28 breaths/min, pulse is 100 beats/min, and her blood pressure is 100/60 mm Hg. You note no jugular vein distention or edema, but do hear crackles and rhonchi. Her urine in the Foley bag is a deep orange color. *What is your impression of the problem?* *(Elicit answers. Discuss the differential diagnosis with the class participants.)*
Slide #27 **Case Study 3 Conclusion** • Mrs. Perkins transported upright on high-flow oxygen. No ALS unit available. • Had leukocytosis and 101.5°F fever, diagnosis of sepsis	Mrs. Perkins was transported upright on high-flow oxygen. No ALS unit was available. She had a fever of 101.5°F and a diagnosis of sepsis. She had a leukocyte count of 14,000 and a chest x-ray consistent with pneumonia. Note the following age-related risk factors for infection:

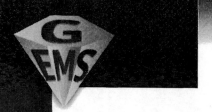

Section 2: Lectures

Slide Text	Additional Information
• Pneumonia confirmed on CXR • Returned to Alzheimer's ward after one week of hospitalization and antibiotics.	decreased pulmonary function, chronic disease and medication use, urinary incontinence, indwelling urinary catheter, and institutional living. Mrs. Perkins was returned to the Alzheimer's ward after one week of hospitalization and antibiotic treatment.

Slide #28
Summary
• Many medical conditions share non-specific symptoms.
• Forming an accurate clinical impression relies on:
  – Keeping high index of suspicion for GI disorders, sepsis, thyroid problems
  – Remaining aware of age-related effects on physiology
  – Considering complications from medications and chronic conditions
	Review slide.

Section 2: Lectures

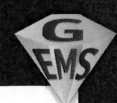

(Optional) Improving Quality of Life

Teaching Tips

This lecture is optional and can be presented if you wish to provide a longer and more comprehensive GEMS course.

This lecture requires some preparation and customization by the Faculty teaching this lecture. Before presenting the lecture, research local community and government resources available to older people in your community. Prepare a handout with this information to pass out during the lecture. Include contact information for your state Ombudsman, Adult Protective Services, and other agencies to which abuse or neglect can be reported. This handout can then be used by providers for referral purposes when on emergency calls with older patients who may need such services. Remember, students are more likely to pass this information along if specific, practical contact information is provided to them during this lecture.

Lecture Outline: Improving Quality of Life

Slide Text	Additional Information
Slide #1 **Improving Quality of Life**	This lecture covers topics found in Chapter 15: Improving Quality of Life. *Before beginning this lecture, catch the class's interest. Tell a story about how EMS improved the quality of an older patient's life.* *Remind students that EMS is the first and sometimes only help available to older patients. A small step that takes only a minute can have a huge positive impact on an older person's life.*
Slide #2 **Objectives** • Discuss the responsibilities of EMS to improve the quality of life of older patients. • Discuss the importance of the social aspect of an older person's life. • Describe how home safety affects quality of life. • Discuss the importance of compassion. • Discuss community strategies for change.	Read objectives.

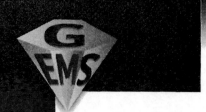

Section 2: Lectures

Slide Text	Additional Information
Slide #3 **Treating Patients as People** • As EMS providers we not only treat patients, but people. • G: Older people have the same concerns, hopes, fears, and interests as other people.	As EMS providers we not only treat patients, but people. Older people have the same concerns, hopes, fears, and interests as other people (consider the "G" in the GEMS diamond). The first lecture in the course discussed attitudes toward older people. Review the perceptions of providers and older people with regard to the role of EMS. These perceptions affect the emergency call and thereby impact the older person's quality of life. For example, communicating in a respectful tone will help the call run more smoothly by helping the patient feel more comfortable. Your actions can have an impact on the quality of life.
Slide #4 **Elements of Quality of Life** • Physical and emotional health • Social connections • Economic security • Safety	Quality of life does not just depend on a person's physical health, but also his or her mental, social, and spiritual well being. These elements will be discussed throughout the lecture. *Explore with the class community, government, and other resources available to older members of the community. Pass out the prepared handout at this point if not done already. (Try to make this relevant to the community in which the students work.)*
Slide #5 **Communication** • Show respect. • Assure patient's privacy. • Explain what is being done. • Allow for patient's input. • Assure patient's dignity.	How you communicate with the patient can have a great impact on the success of the call physically and emotionally. When communicating, show respect by using "Mr.," "Mrs.," or a professional title they have earned such as "Reverend," "Sister," or "Dr.," and the patient's last name. Even if the patient is unconscious, communicate in a respectful way. The patient may be able to perceive what is happening. Privacy can be very important to older people. If the patient lives in a facility, try to find a private space to talk with the patient if possible. When

Section 2: Lectures

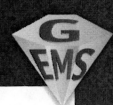

Slide Text	Additional Information
	conducting the exam, only expose the part of the body being examined at that time, to help preserve privacy and warmth.
	Explain to the patient what is being done, and allow patient input. These are small steps you can take that will make a big difference to the patient. Older patients have as much of a right to know what you are doing to them as younger patients do.
	Obtain input from the patient. Gentle questioning may reveal additional information critical to the call, but that you may not obtain if the patient feels uncomfortable with you.
	Taking these steps will help assure the patient's dignity.
Slide #6 **Health Care Assessment** • What does the patient consider the primary health concern(s)? • Does the patient have a doctor? • Does the patient feel he/she currently has the right amount of medical attention?	You can get an idea of a patient's quality of life from the way he or she answers questions during the emergency call. For example, a negative answer to the question "Do you feel you have the right amount of medical attention?" would indicate that the patient may need a referral to obtain better health care. When talking with an older patient, remember to be aware of nonverbal communication. This can provide additional clues beyond what the patient tells you.
Slide #7 **Nutrition and Hydration Assessment** • Does the patient live alone? • **E:** Check the freezer, refrigerator, and cupboards. • Are meals brought in? • **E:** Ask the patient what was eaten at his or her last meal.	Inadequate nutrition and hydration can cause physical and mental problems in older patients due to changes with age. Assess the environment for signs of poor nutrition (consider the "E" in the GEMS diamond). *Again, discuss community, government, and other resources that might be accessed to help older people obtain access to better nutrition and hydration. For example, does a local church provide such a service?*

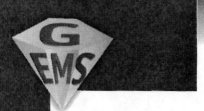

Section 2: Lectures

Slide Text	Additional Information
Slide #8 **Assessing Social Connections** • Does the patient live alone? • Is there family nearby? • Is there someone you can call for the patient? • Does someone visit to help the patient? • Does the patient have someone to call for help?	Connections with other people are important. Isolation and loneliness can have a negative affect on an older person's health. Ask questions such as: • Does someone live here with you? • Do you have family nearby? • Is there someone you would like me to call? • Does someone come in to help you? • Do you have friends you can call on if you need help? Keep in mind that the patient may not answer these questions accurately if he or she feels embarrassed, ashamed, or defensive. An angry or elusive "yes" response can indicate that the real answer is "no." Remember to observe for nonverbal elements of communication. If you determine that the patient has few social connections, a referral may be in order. Provide the older person with information on community resources if appropriate. Remember the "S" in the GEMS diamond.
Slide #9 **Assessing Economic Security** • Is the home in good repair? • Are the utilities functional? • Do appliances work? • Is the home too warm or too cool?	Factors such as an environment that is in disrepair may indicate economic difficulties. Are there immediate health or safety concerns present? Asking the patient these questions can be difficult and may require delicacy. Your local Area Agencies on Aging can help older people find solutions to a variety of problems, including economic ones. These agencies have senior information programs that track all resources in the community. Nutrition programs, transportation services, and senior centers are some of the resources that may be available in your community. Remember the "E" in the GEMS diamond.

Section 2: Lectures

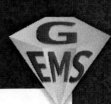

Slide Text	Additional Information
Slide #10 **Assessing the Living Environment** • Is this a safe environment? • Is there adequate food in the home? • Is it sanitary? • Is this environment supportive of the resident's needs?	Safety is important for older patients, who are at an increased risk for injury due to the physical changes with age discussed in Lecture 2. How immediate are the concerns? *Review with the students your area's local resources for addressing safety hazards. Do they know how to access emergency resources after normal business hours?* If you note safety hazards, explain these hazards to the patient and suggest modifications that can be made to remove the hazard. Refer to Appendix C in the textbook for an extensive home safety checklist.
Slide #11 **The EMS Provider as an Advocate** *What is the reasonable extent of your role as an advocate for your older patients?*	Considering the class discussion so far, discuss with the class the opportunities afforded them as advocates. What is the reasonable extent of their role as an advocate?
Slide #12 **Case Study** • Dispatched to an assisted-living residence • 86-year-old Mr. Sanchez has altered level of consciousness • E: Four residents are housed in two bedrooms.	You are dispatched to an assisted-living residence for an 86-year-old man, Mr. Sanchez, with an altered level of consciousness. You arrive to a single-story private residence where four people are housed in two bedrooms and movement is greatly compromised (consider the "E" in the GEMS diamond). Although medication charts are kept, they have not been updated in the last 36 hours. No additional records are available. Your patient appears confused and cannot remember recent events. You must ask him each question several times and he repeatedly asks who you are. *Discuss resources in your community that could be accessed in this case.*
Slide #13 **Case Study (continued)** • Home is uncomfortably cool. • Staff has little information. • You observe clutter, fire code violations.	You note that the home is uncomfortably cool. The staff has little information on the residents. You also observe clutter and several fire code violations (consider the "E" in the GEMS diamond).

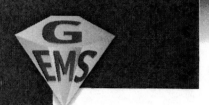

Section 2: Lectures

Slide Text	Additional Information
	Are there legal, regulatory, or licensing issues in this situation? *With the class, attempt to come to an agreement on an action plan relevant to this situation.*
Slide #14 **Case Study Conclusion** • Mr. Sanchez transported to local ED without incident • Situation reported to state Ombudsman, Adult Protective Services, Fire Marshal's office • Issues could not be resolved. • Remaining patients were relocated.	Upon arrival, the staff is unable to advise as to why EMS was called. The staff member who called 9-1-1 is off duty and has left work. Patient records are not available to the staff, and the manager will not be back until several days later. Every state has an Ombudsman who is responsible for reviewing and resolving complaints in nursing homes and other long-term care facilities. EMS contacted the state Ombudsman, Adult Protective Services, and the Fire Marshal's office to report what they found on this emergency call. *Provide students with contact information for their state Ombudsman, Adult Protective Services, and/or other agency to which suspected abuse or neglect can be reported.*
Slide # 15 **Summary** • The EMS provider can make a difference. • When assessing the patient, consider quality of life issues. • Access resources. • Be an advocate.	*Review slide.* *Remind students that their role goes beyond that of a clinician. Reinforce opportunities for advocacy and responsibilities in relation to the older patient's quality of life.*

Scenarios

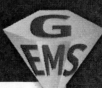

Section 3

Stephen H. Thomas, MD, MPH

Contents

- **Scenarios Overview** 148
- **BLS Scenarios** 149
    - Communication Challenges 149
    - Do Not Resuscitate Orders 152
    - Stroke 154
    - Medication Interactions 157
    - Elder Abuse and Neglect 160
    - Delirium vs. Dementia 163
- **ALS Scenarios** 166
    - Communication Challenges 166
    - Do Not Resuscitate Orders 170
    - Stroke 172
    - Medication Interactions 175
    - Elder Abuse and Neglect 179
    - Delirium vs. Dementia 182

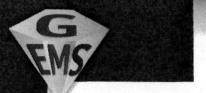

Section 3: Scenarios

Scenarios Overview

The scenario component of the GEMS course is designed to promote case-based learning through small group discussion. The GEMS Faculty will present a case and provide initial information that would be available to EMS providers on arrival at the scene. The students then work through the case as a team, requesting information from the Faculty and proposing management strategies. Students should be allowed to work through the scenario as a group. The Faculty should take a passive role until the group has met an impassable point or to help summarize or emphasize important points.

During the course:

- At the beginning of the day during registration, assign a group number to each individual. This number will be used later to efficiently organize the students into their skill station and scenario groups.
- When it is time to begin the first scenario session, divide the students into smaller groups for instruction according to the group numbers assigned to them during registration. Assign each group to one of the smaller breakout rooms.

The materials for each scenario are as follows:

Case Presentation

Both BLS and ALS cases are provided. Select the appropriate case for your audience. Read the initial information as written to introduce the case.

Faculty Information

Use this information to answer students' questions, to stimulate discussion, or to provide additional information. It is not necessary to present all of the Faculty information. It should be revealed selectively.

Management Strategies

Pose these questions to the group during the active "case management" or after the scenario has been completed.

Issues in Management

Highlight the management issues during "case management" or after the scenario has been completed. *Note that both appropriate management techniques, and pitfalls to avoid, are addressed.*

Core Knowledge Points

Stimulate further case discussion by highlighting the key points about the case, including pathophysiological principles and a more complete discussion of management issues.

Case Development

Provide additional information on the progression of the case, patient status, and appropriate BLS and ALS interventions after initial assessment and management strategies have been discussed. *Local protocols should be addressed throughout the scenario. Faculty should have a working knowledge of the local or state protocols for the scenario that they are teaching.*

Summary

Share the major points of emphasis with the students at the end of the case.

Section 3: Scenarios

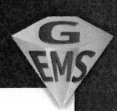

BLS Scenarios: Communication Challenges

The scenarios portion of the concurrent skill/scenario station on Communication and Assessment is 45 minutes long and designed to cover two scenarios. When you are finished discussing this scenario, move on to the ALS communication scenario on page 166. These scenarios are applicable to both BLS and ALS audiences.

This case is designed to facilitate discussion on the importance of communication with the older patient. The patient is stable with a history of a previous CVA and has a hard time with verbal communications. Discussion should be centered on other types of communication with patients who have trouble communicating; however, clinical aspects of the scenario are also discussed.

■ Objectives

At the completion of this scenario, the student will be able to:
- Analyze the needs of an older patient with sensory deficits.
- Formulate a plan to better communicate with an older patient with sensory deficits.

■ Case Presentation

You are dispatched to the home of an 80-year-old man who has activated his medic alert system, indicating that he needs an ambulance response. There was no other information available at the time of your dispatch. You arrive at the house and find the door locked, but you are able to gain entry through a back door near the kitchen. As you enter the house, you find the patient incoherent on the kitchen floor. He appears to be agitated.

■ Faculty Information

Initial assessment
ABCDEs:
- Airway: The patient appears to have an open airway and there are no problems handling secretions, but you are unable to confirm airway patency by listening to the patient speak—he does not appear to be following your instructions.
- Breathing: The patient has a respiratory rate of 14 breaths/min and there is good chest rise, with normal bilaterally equal breath sounds.
- Circulation: The patient's blood pressure is 140/82 mmHg and the heart rate is 72 beats/min and irregular. The extremities appear to be warm and well perfused and the pulses are normal.
- Disability: The patient appears to be awake and alert, but he is unable to give a history. At times, he appears to be attempting to talk but no history is obtainable. He is moving both arms with good strength but is lying on the floor and does not appear able to move the right leg.
- Exposure: There do not appear to be signs of trauma on the patient's head, chest, or abdomen. He is not wearing any medic alert jewelry.

ALS Information:
- Pulse Ox: 97%
- ECG: Atrial fibrillation
- Blood sugar: 112 mg/dL

SAMPLE History:
- Signs: He has tenderness on the right hip area when this region is palpated.
- Allergies: When the patient is asked questions, he looks at the provider who is asking the questions but does not verbalize any answers.
- Medications: Same as above
- Past history: Same as above
- Last meal: Same as above
- Events leading up: Same as above, but you notice a chair turned over, suggesting he may have fallen.

GEMS diamond:
- G: Patient is attempting to talk, but is unable.
- E: A chair is turned over, suggesting he may have fallen.
- M: Patient is unable to give a history.
- S: Patient appears to live alone.

The patient's presentation suggests having fallen down as a result of either syncope or a mechanical (eg, slip-and-fall) problem. The patient appears to be alert and awake, and there are signs of a right hip injury, but the patient is nonverbal.

Management Strategies

What are the immediate priorities for this patient?
- The first priority for this and any patient is the airway. There should be some concerns about the airway due to the patient's inability to talk. Inability to talk can indicate a foreign body obstruction or similar mechanical problem. Investigate this in the physical examination. However, the lack of respiratory distress suggests that complete obstruction is not the cause for this patient's nonverbal status.
- The second priority for this patient is to determine, if possible, whether any other life-threatening injuries were sustained as a result of the fall. The overall assessment of the patient's physical condition does not indicate this, although there are physical findings that suggest a hip fracture.
- Another priority for the patient is to determine the reason for his fall, and if this dictates any emergency intervention. For example, the patient could have had a hypoglycemic event with a subsequent fall, and he may still be hypoglycemic. This would be an example of a metabolic problem which could also explain his inability to give a history.

Can the patient be moved after the initial assessment?
- When there are no signs of particularly concerning trauma, and airway and oxygen concerns have been met, additional aspects of the evaluation can proceed with the patient on a stretcher. This may enhance the patient's comfort, allow the patient to be in a position to communicate better, and allow transportation to take place if the situation requires.

Issues in Management
- This patient appears to have had a syncopal or mechanical fall and sustained a hip fracture, activating his medical alert system when he was unable to get up. At this point, due to his nonverbal status, you cannot obtain the history surrounding his fall and pertinent current complaints.
- However, the patient appears to be alert and has no signs that indicate a mechanical obstruction of the airway. You should consider that the patient's communication issues may be unrelated to his acute presentation.
- Consider alternatives to verbal communication in order to obtain a history from nonverbal patients.

Core Knowledge Points

What are some explanations for patients being nonverbal, and yet apparently awake and alert?
- Metabolic issues could cause patients to appear awake and alert, and yet have neurologic alterations that make them nonverbal. Similarly, mass lesions in the brain or mass lesions or foreign bodies in the airway tract could result in patients being alert but nonverbal. In patients who have stable vital signs, however, and appear to be neurologically normal other than nonverbal status, the likelihood of these explanations decreases.

Section 3: Scenarios

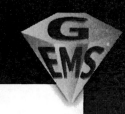

- Patients can be apparently nonverbal for reasons other than acute medical events. Examples include the following:
  1. *Previous stroke.* Patients are continually getting better stroke care, and stroke survival and outcomes are likely to continue to improve. One result is that EMS providers will encounter more patients who have had strokes. You should not be surprised to encounter patients who have aphasia and thus have a chronic inability to verbalize complaints, as in this scenario. Overall, a previous stroke may be the most likely explanation for the current presentation.
  2. *Language barriers.* Patients with language barriers will generally not be totally nonverbal, as in this scenario, but be aware that patients who don't understand or speak English may appear to have a neurologic deficit (eg, aphasia), when in fact there is no such deficit. You would expect patients with language barriers to talk—albeit in a language other than English—but patients may be confused, anxious, and unable to understand that questions are being asked.
  3. *Anxiety.* Patients who are very anxious may be too upset or distraught to effectively communicate. You would not expect such patients to be nonverbal, but in some cases patients who are anxious can have a surprisingly difficult time explaining their symptoms.
  4. *Tracheostomy patients.* Patients who have tracheostomies may not have the attachments in place which allow them to phonate. Such patients will usually be easily identified by visualization of their neck tracheostomy site, but sometimes the tracheostomy may not be immediately obvious.

How can EMS providers improve communications with nonverbal patients?
- Patients who have had strokes in the past and are therefore nonverbal may have medic alert bracelets identifying them. Written communication may be possible, depending on the level of the patient's stroke and whether or not writing abilities were affected. It is worth trying some note writing to see if these patients are able to communicate this way.
- Communication with patients who have language barriers may be facilitated with family or acquaintances who can help translate. Sometimes a neighbor is a good resource.
- Patients who are anxious may respond to calming. Incoherent, ineffective speech may then become easier to understand, making a history obtainable.
- Patients who have tracheostomies and who are unable to talk may be able to communicate by writing, and may be able to indicate the location of the appropriate tracheostomy equipment.

■ Case Development

With a pencil and paper, the patient is able to indicate that he has had an old stroke and, as an old problem, has difficulty talking. He uses nonverbal communication such as head nodding and writing to indicate that he simply tripped and was unable to get up, thereby needing his medic alert system for assistance. The patient is transported to the hospital, where he is found to have a hip fracture with no other injuries, and no change in his baseline neurologic status.

■ Summary

Patients who are unable to give a history may have chronic problems rather than acute issues responsible for inability to communicate. These patients may be able to give history using other (nonverbal) means, such as pen and paper. Given the improved treatment and survival from stroke, you may commonly encounter stroke survivors with communication difficulties. Stroke patients are also likely to have other problems, such as falls, and thus are more likely to interact with EMS. While balancing the needs of a good history with those of avoiding protracted transport delays, attempt to use nonverbal means to obtain history from all apparently nonverbal patients.

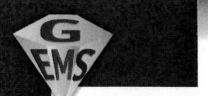

Section 3: Scenarios

BLS Scenarios: Do Not Resuscitate Orders

Note to Faculty: Because of differences in local protocols, this scenario requires some customization. Before the course, prepare samples of valid DNR orders to show students, and also bring documents that are not valid per your local protocol.

This case is designed to facilitate discussion on do not resuscitate (DNR) orders. The patient is in cardiac arrest upon arrival and requires no care. Discussion should include local protocols regarding DNR orders and what must be done to honor them. Advance directives should also be discussed.

▪ Objectives

At the completion of this scenario, the student will be able to:
- Recognize a valid DNR order in their local jurisdiction.
- Identify the wishes of a patient with a DNR order.
- Explain the psychological impact of sudden stressors on both family and EMS providers.

▪ Case Presentation

You are dispatched to the home of a 74-year-old female cancer patient who has disseminated liver cancer and has been discharged home for comfort care measures. Family members state that the patient was having a hard time breathing and they activated 9-1-1, because they didn't want to see her suffering. When you arrive at the patient's side, it is clear that the patient has expired. There are no signs of life, but the patient is warm and there are no signs of dependent lividity or rigor mortis. The patient has a DNR that is valid in your jurisdiction (document and/or bracelet).

▪ Faculty Information

This patient's assessment shows her to be dead. No resuscitation is indicated, as there is a valid DNR. The clinical picture is one of a DNR patient with end-stage disease who has died at home, with EMS activated by family members who were basically not sure what else to do.

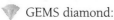 GEMS diamond:
- G: Patient has disseminated liver cancer and is home for comfort care measures.
- E: Nothing noted.
- M: None noted.
- S: The family is distraught.

As an experienced provider, you are working with a new BLS provider who has not yet seen a patient die. This new provider behaves professionally at the scene but is clearly emotionally impacted by the fact that he has been asked not to care for a deceased patient. The distraught family members at the scene have also affected him.

▪ Management Strategies

Should this patient undergo resuscitation?
- The patient had a valid DNR and is in full cardiorespiratory arrest with no signs of life and pupils fixed and dilated. There are no heart tones or breath sounds. The ECG shows asystole. There is no indication for resuscitation.

Note to Faculty: At this point, hold a discussion regarding the local protocol regarding DNR in your area. Show the samples of valid DNR orders and documents that are not valid per your local protocol. Have students review the forms and assess whether or not they are valid. Ensure that by the end of this session, the students know what is accepted as a valid DNR order per your local protocol.

Section 3: Scenarios

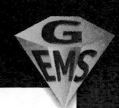

Since the patient has a DNR order in force, the management strategies for this particular scenario revolve around "non-medical" issues.
- ALS and BLS priorities are similar.
- Though no medical treatment is indicated, there are important interventions and interactions for EMS providers at a scene such as this.

Should this BLS provider be told to "just deal with it?"
- This provider has experienced a distressing event and may not know how to deal with the emotions that are being experienced. Encouraging your partner to talk about his or her feelings following a bad call can be the first step towards decreasing the stress.

Should this BLS provider be assessed by mental health professionals?
- EMS providers occasionally experience situations that cause powerful emotional reactions well beyond the norm. These incidents can produce acute stress reactions. Some providers will be able to find outlets to relieve these stresses; however, others will not. In many areas, CISM teams are available to assist with coping. Mental health workers are also available for the providers who, after CISM intervention, continue to experience ongoing stress.

What are some of the signs of increased distress following an incident?
- Providers can experience many reactions. These include: difficulty making decisions, angry outbursts, extreme hyperactivity, difficulty sleeping or nightmares, panic attacks, and decreased alertness to surroundings. There are also more subtle signs that may be noted if you are familiar with the provider. These include excessive smoking, increased or decreased food intake, excessive humor, or silence. In EMS, it is important to look out for each other.

■ Issues in Management
- Even with the knowledge that their loved one has a terminal illness, the patient's death will frequently pose a crisis for family members. This is understandable, and providers should have patience with the family members and attempt to help with whatever arrangements they can.
- Your management of this situation should also include debriefing with the newer crew member. While the priorities at the scene for this case are similar to those in other DNR situations, the added factor in this scenario is the fact that the newer providers needs should be addressed with critical incident stress management (CISM).
- CISM is an important part of dealing with the death that is encountered on an all-too-frequent basis in emergency care of the older patient. EMS providers may attempt to bury feelings of emotional concern over the death of an older patient and/or DNR patient deaths, as these deaths may seem more "expected" than other deaths (eg, pediatric trauma patients), which "more understandably" cause emotional reaction. CISM should always be considered in a case such as this.

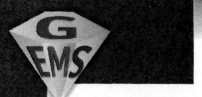

Section 3: Scenarios

BLS Scenarios: Stroke

This case is designed to facilitate discussion on care of the older patient with a CVA. The patient is unstable with a recent history of an embolic stroke. Discussion should be centered on the management and transport of the older patient who has experienced a stroke.

■ Objectives

At the completion of this scenario, the student will be able to:
- Recognize the signs and symptoms of an older patient experiencing a possible stroke.
- Determine the proper treatment for an older patient experiencing a possible stroke.
- Recall the need to determine the time of onset of symptoms when completing the patient history.

■ Case Presentation

You are dispatched to the home of a 75-year-old woman whose family reports that she has had difficulty speaking and walking for the past 30 minutes.

The patient's daughter states that she was talking with her mother this morning and she suddenly started slurring her words. The daughter was going to take her mother to the hospital, but she could not get her up to walk to the car.

■ Faculty Information

Initial Assessment
ABCDEs:
- Airway: Open, the patient has no problems handling secretions.
- Breathing: Respiratory rate is 14 breaths/min with good chest rise and bilateral breath sounds.
- Circulation: Blood pressure is 140/80 mm Hg, heart rate is 68 beats/min, the skin is warm and well perfused, and distal pulses are normal.
- Disability: The patient is conscious and alert but has garbled speech and has significant weakness in the right arm and right leg.
- Exposure: There are no signs of trauma to the patient's head or the remainder of her body, but right-sided facial droop is noted.

ALS Information:
- ECG: Normal sinus rhythm
- Blood sugar: 124 mg/dL
- 12-lead ECG: Atrial fibrillation with no signs of ischemia

SAMPLE History:
- Signs: Slurred speech, weakness to the right arm and leg, right-sided facial droop
- Allergies: Denied by the daughter
- Medications: The daughter states that the patient has only irregularly taken her Coumadin therapy.
- Past history: The daughter is able to give the patient's past medical history, which includes atrial fibrillation.
- Last meal: Lunch 2 hours earlier
- Event leading up: The patient's daughter called EMS when she was speaking with her mother and the mother had a sudden change in speech pattern, accompanied by weakness. The patient did not fall and there is no history of trauma.

▼ GEMS diamond:
- G: Patient has garbled speech and significant weakness in the right arm and right leg, history of atrial fibrillation.
- E: Nothing noted.
- M: Daughter states that patient only irregularly takes Coumadin therapy.
- S: Patient's daughter is on-scene and willing to help.

Section 3: Scenarios

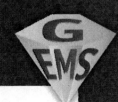

This patient, with no history of trauma, has a clinical picture consistent with acute stroke. The past medical history makes it relatively likely that this stroke is due to a clot.

Management Strategies

What is the patient's neurologic status?
- It is not always necessary to assign ratings with various stroke scales; sometimes it is best to simply describe what you saw when interacting with the patient. In this case, the fact that the patient is unable to speak clearly and has obvious right upper and lower extremity weakness is probably sufficient history for a receiving hospital emergency physician to make arrangements appropriate for stroke team evaluation.
- There are several prehospital stroke scales in use in the U.S. The Cincinnati Prehospital Stroke Scale evaluates for facial droop, arm drift, or abnormal speech; if any one of those three signs is abnormal, then the patient is at high risk of having a stroke. A slightly more complicated stroke screen, the Los Angeles Prehospital Stroke Screen, is in use in other EMS systems. The Los Angeles Prehospital Stroke Screen takes into account the patient's age, history of seizures, symptom duration, baseline ambulatory status, glucose level, and any other obvious asymmetry and facial smile, grip, or arm strength; its goal is to identify patients who may have strokes requiring urgent care in the receiving hospital emergency department. EMS providers should use whichever stroke scale is in use in their own system. *Note to Faculty: Review the stroke scale used in your local protocol.*

What are your initial management (treatment) priorities?
- **BLS treatment priorities:**
  1. Obtain a history of the deficits. As important as describing the deficits is noting the time of onset.
  2. The patient should be monitored for deterioration, and appropriate therapy (eg, airway control) started if such deterioration occurs.
  3. Transport and/or assist ALS providers.

Note to Faculty: Discuss the following only if you are using this scenario with an ALS audience. Skip this part when discussing with a BLS audience.
- **ALS treatment priorities:**
  1. BLS priorities, plus provide advanced airway if the patient's airway deteriorates.
  2. Check blood sugar and treat if low.
  3. Attempt intravenous access en route to the emergency department.
  4. In appropriate jurisdictions, notify the receiving hospital of the impending arrival of a patient with a suspected stroke.

Issues in Management

- Stroke patients should be given oxygen.
- Vital signs should be measured frequently.
- A general medical assessment should include investigation for signs of trauma, cardiovascular abnormalities, and neurologic changes such as ocular signs or symptoms, level of consciousness, Glasgow Coma Scale, limb movements, and meningeal signs.
- One of the most important things for definitive stroke therapy (thrombolysis or fibrinolysis) decision-making is to determine when the patient was "last seen normal." This is because of the relatively narrow thrombolytic window—three hours for IV lysis. Because of this narrow window, rapid EMS evaluation and transport are paramount in patients with suspected stroke.

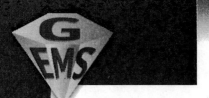

Section 3: Scenarios

▪ Case Development
The patient's situation remains unchanged during transport. There is no neurologic deterioration. Vital signs remain stable and unchanged. The patient is still unable to talk or give a history.

▪ Management Strategies
What are your management and treatment priorities now?
- Since this patient is stable, there is little further active intervention required in the prehospital setting. It is important, however, to ensure documentation of when patients were last seen normal, and if possible to bring patients' family members or caregivers to the ED so a definitive history can be immediately given. This minimizes delay during stroke team evaluation.

▪ Core Knowledge Points
Which patients are most likely to have strokes that can be treated with definitive therapy?
- Patients who experience a stroke due to a clot, or embolic stroke, are candidates for thrombolytic or "clot-busting" therapy. This case involves a patient with atrial fibrillation, which is a known risk factor for development of embolic disease. Patients who experienced trauma or who have severe headache are less likely to have embolic stroke and more likely to have hematomas or subarachnoid hemorrhage.

What should EMS providers do in evaluating and managing stroke patients?
- Standard evaluation of the patient should include current presentation and past medical history. The past medical history can both provide information relevant to stroke diagnosis, and also begin to address potential contraindications to definitive (thrombolytic) therapy.
- Patients should be assessed for signs of trauma. This could be either the cause of the apparent stroke, or trauma can occur as a result of a stroke-related fall.
- Other than supportive measures, such as airway and hemodynamic support as indicated, perhaps the most important thing to do is to rapidly evaluate the patient's neurologic condition, determine when the patient was last seen normal (ie, at their baseline), and transport the patient as rapidly as possible. Stroke therapy is time-critical, and in the absence of a definitive history of time of onset, most hospitals will not be able to provide thrombolytic therapy. Therefore, obtaining and documenting information as to when patients were last seen normal is very important.
- Some local EMS systems use prehospital stroke scales. Examples of these are the Cincinnati and the Los Angeles scales discussed earlier. The EMS provider should use whichever stroke scale is used and recommended locally; check local protocol.
- In many cities, receiving hospitals have established stroke teams who are specially trained to rapidly mobilize and evaluate patients with suspected stroke in the ED. These teams, instituted due to the time-critical nature of acute stroke evaluation, are activated by prehospital radio contact with the receiving ED in most places. Therefore, in EMS systems where this is relevant, notifying the receiving hospital of the impending arrival of a patient with an acute stroke should be a high priority. Detailed information is not necessary; the simple data that a patient with an acute stroke will be arriving, and the time of symptom duration, provide a minimum amount of crucial data.

▪ Summary
Acute stroke is becoming an area of intense interest both in the hospital and prehospital settings. Your role in rapid identification of patients eligible for definitive therapy (thrombolysis now, with other potential therapies still under investigation) is a vital one. Given the high incidence of acute stroke in the older population, and the potential benefits for definitive therapy, you can play an important role in getting vital information and rapidly transporting patients to appropriate stroke care centers.

Section 3: Scenarios

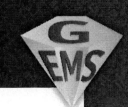

BLS Scenarios: Medication Interactions

This case is designed to facilitate discussion on the importance of medication history and common medication problems. The patient is in profound bradycardia but otherwise stable, with a recent history of a near syncopal event and weakness from recent medication changes. Discussion should be centered on the clinical assessment of the weakness and the importance of obtaining a complete medication history.

■ Objectives
At the completion of this scenario, the student will be able to:
- Determine the need to obtain a complete medication history for the older patient.
- Specify the components of a complete medication history.
- Formulate a plan to evaluate the older patient with a complaint related to a medication reaction.

■ Case Presentation
You are dispatched to the home of a 70-year-old man who has had a near syncopal event while walking from his bedroom to the kitchen. The patient is in his bed at home, has no chest pain, and notes that he feels "very tired." The patient's daughter and primary caregiver states that the patient saw his doctor two days ago.

■ Faculty Information
Initial Assessment
ABCDEs:
- Airway: Open, no signs of obstruction.
- Breathing: Respiratory rate 16 breaths/min with good breath sounds and adequate chest rise; SpO_2 is 98% on room air.
- Circulation: Heart rate is 32 beats/min; skin is pale and slightly cool; blood pressure is 120/80 mm Hg.
- Disability: The patient has spontaneous eye opening and is conversant with no signs of disability.
- Exposure: There are no signs of trauma on inspection of the patient.

SAMPLE History:
- Signs: Patient feels very tired.
- Allergies: Penicillin
- Medications: Aspirin, nitro-patch, digoxin, and furosemide (all prescribed by his regular physician) digoxin (Lanoxin) prescribed by his cardiologist.
- Past history: Angina, atrial fibrillation, and CHF
- Last meal: Dinner 2 hours ago
- Events leading up: Hasn't been feeling well for last two days

ALS Information:
- ECG: Atrial fibrillation
- Blood sugar: 108 mg/dL

GEMS diamond:
- G: Patient has no chest pain and feels very tired. History of angina, atrial fibrillation, CHF.
- E: Nothing noted.
- M: Patient takes aspirin, digoxin, furosemide (prescribed by Dr. Jones), and Lanoxin (prescribed by Dr. Bartlett), and has a nitro patch. Daughter states patient was placed on new medication (Lanoxin) by cardiologist two days ago and hasn't been feeling well since.
- S: Daughter is patient's primary caregiver.

The patient has evidence of significant bradycardia.

Section 3: Scenarios

■ Management Strategies

Based on this patient's presentation, what are the likely causes of the bradycardia?
- Acute coronary syndrome
- Medication/toxicologic considerations

What is your general impression?
- The patient is bradycardic but has an acceptable blood pressure.

What are your initial treatment priorities?
- BLS treatment priorities:
  1. As stabilization and transport continue, obtain a more complete history.
  2. Maintain the airway and apply oxygen.
  3. Monitor blood pressure.
  4. Rapid transport and/or assist ALS providers
  5. Monitor heart rate and appearance of new symptoms.

Note to Faculty: Discuss the following only if you are using this scenario with an ALS audience. Skip this part when discussing with a BLS audience.
- ALS treatment priorities:
  1. BLS priorities, plus consider advanced airway maneuvers if the patient situation deteriorates
  2. Attempt intravenous access on the way to the emergency department.
  3. Cautious fluid resuscitation while monitoring patient's breath sounds.
  4. Consider pharmacologic (eg, atropine) or electrical management of patient's bradycardia if necessary.
  5. Provide treatment appropriate for possible acute coronary syndrome (aspirin, nitroglycerin and/or morphine sulfate if there is no hypotension, oxygen).
  6. Ongoing ECG monitoring with a 12-lead ECG if available.

■ Issues in Management

- This patient is stable but has significant bradycardia. The goal for management of patients with profound bradycardia is to address the patient's symptoms and hemodynamic status. Care should be taken to not stress the patient's cardiovascular status. The patient should remain in a supine position, and not be asked to stand or walk. In this particular case, the patient has a heart rate in the 30s, which is significantly depressed, but there is no hemodynamic concern and there are no other indications for immediate treatment of the heart rate outlined in ACLS.
- The fact that no specific therapy is indicated does not mean that you cannot fulfill an important role in evaluation of the patient. In this particular instance, the history is the key aspect for prehospital management. The patient's family member, who notes that the patient had recently started a new prescription, may or may not be available to the evaluating physicians at the receiving emergency department, so be sure to obtain as much information as possible.

■ Core Knowledge Points

What is the effect of medications on the older population?
- Medication effects on the older patient can be similar to their effects in younger patients, but in some cases (especially when there is limited reserve in a system such as the cardiovascular system) older people may be more predisposed to having side effects from medications. This is obviously a particular concern when multiple medications are being taken, which may have synergistic effects in producing side effects.
- Older patients are frequently on multiple medications; various studies suggest that on average, older people are on at least three to four different medications simultaneously, and in some cases many more. With multiple medications and their potential interactions, older people are particularly predisposed to experiencing drug interactions.

Section 3: Scenarios

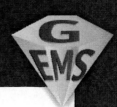

- The fact that the patient recently started a new prescription and then became symptomatic could suggest that this prescription was the cause. When asked, the family volunteers that the patient felt different since he started the new medication. This information, critical to the appropriate evaluation of the cause of the patient's bradycardia, was offered by the family upon direct questioning.

Why should you focus on getting an accurate history?
- EMS providers have access to those who know patients best when they respond to the patient's home. These family members are often the caregivers for the patient and they may not be able to make it to the evaluating emergency department in time to provide useful information to the emergency department staff. Therefore, you are in an unusually advantageous position to get a useful history from multiple family members and/or caregivers. In a case such as this one, obtaining this history allowed for the rapid diagnosis of the patient's bradycardia at the receiving institution.

How should you deal with potential medication interactions in older patients?
- The best thing to do, besides getting a list of medications, is to actually bring the medications into the hospital with the patient. This fact, critical to the outcome of this particular case, allows the receiving emergency physicians to know which medications the patient is on, and know their doses and dosing intervals. Even if the medications are not related to the patient's presentation, this information allows appropriate medicines to be administered to the patient at the hospital should admission be required. In this particular case, the cardiologist was unaware that the patient was already taking digoxin under the direction of his primary care physician, and prescribed Lanoxin, another form of digoxin. Upon further questioning, the family related that the patient had only seen his cardiologist once before and that his family doctor had provided all his other prescriptions.

Case Development

This 70-year-old man had near-syncope related to bradycardia. The patient had recently started a new prescription of a similar medication. During transport, no intervention was required, but the patient did have a critical EMS intervention in EMS bringing the medications to the receiving hospital.

Summary

Patients with bradycardia do not always require medical management, but there are other prehospital interventions which may be important.
- Older patients are often on multiple medications. These medications are sometimes prescribed by different physicians, who may not have complete knowledge of other medications the patient is taking. Multiple medications may interact, causing an emergency. Always identify all medications (both prescription and herbal/nontraditional), and bring the actual medication bottles to the receiving facility with the patient.
- This particular patient's bradycardia was due to the combined effect of the patient's Lanoxin and the digoxin. Such an interaction would likely have occurred in a younger patient, but the older patient who has a reduced cardiovascular reserve is particularly susceptible to this type of side effect.
- As an EMS provider, you have access to family members and other caregivers who may not make it to the hospital in time to pass along vital history. Speak with these family members and caregivers to get critical aspects of the history. You are also well positioned to advocate with the family to make sure that all the patient's physicians are aware of the patient's complete medication regimen.

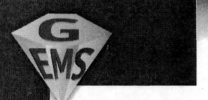

Section 3: Scenarios

BLS Scenarios: Elder Abuse and Neglect

This case is designed to facilitate discussion on elder abuse and maltreatment. The patient is stable with arm pain from a stated fall, but evidence of additional abuse is present throughout the assessment. Discussion should be centered on elder abuse and maltreatment. Local protocols on reporting requirements should be reviewed.

■ Objectives

At the completion of this scenario, the student will be able to:
- Explain the common signs and symptoms attributed to elder abuse.
- Discuss the requirements for reporting suspected elder abuse.
- Describe the signs and symptoms of neglect.

■ Case Presentation

You are dispatched to a home where a 50-year-old man is caring for his 80-year-old father and called 9-1-1. The man states that his father fell and hurt his arm this evening. He wants you to take his father to the emergency department for an X-ray.

■ Faculty Information

Initial Assessment
ABCDEs:
- Airway: The airway is open and the patient has no problems handling secretions; he is conversing.
- Breathing: The respiratory rate is 16 breaths/min and there is good chest rise and bilateral breath sounds. SpO_2 is 97% on room air.
- Circulation: The patient's blood pressure is 160/90 mm Hg with a heart rate of 90 beats/min. The skin is warm and well perfused, and distal pulses are normal.
- Disability: The patient is conscious and alert and has a pain-related weakness in the right upper extremity.
- Exposure: You note multiple contusions in the chest and abdomen. The contusions range from a violet to a yellow greenish hue. There are no signs of head trauma.

SAMPLE History:
- Signs: Patient complains of right arm pain.
- Allergies: Denied
- Medications: Aspirin, Xanax
- Past history: Takes Xanax for trouble sleeping
- Last meal: Dinner 3 hours ago
- Events leading up: Son states that his father fell.

ALS Information:
- The ECG shows normal sinus rhythm and blood sugar is 124 mg/dL.

GEMS diamond:
- G: Trauma noted.
- E: Nothing noted.
- M: Patient takes aspirin, Xanax.
- S: Son states that father fell, wants EMS providers to transport patient to hospital for an x-ray. Additional bruising is noted. Son interrupts and answers for father, stating that father is clumsy and often falls. Patient does not interject.

The patient's son is the person who activated EMS. The son tells EMS that the patient fell on his right arm. When EMS providers attempt to question the patient about the circumstances of the fall, or of the other bruising that is noted, the patient's son interrupts and answers the questions. The son states that his father is clumsy and often falls. After the first few questions where the son takes over providing the history, the patient does not attempt to correct his son or interject. When asked if the history provided by the son is correct or if he has anything to add, the patient just shakes his head.

Section 3: Scenarios

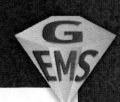

■ Management Strategies

What is this patient's management priority?
- The patient has a complaint of right upper extremity injury. Since distal pulses are intact and the patient is able to use the extremity, but with some pain on range of motion, the injury is very unlikely to be limb threatening.
- There is bruising on the patient's chest and abdomen which does not appear to be associated with acutely life-threatening injuries. The various color shades of the bruising indicates that some of these bruises are old, and should therefore not be an acute threat to the patient's health. This is reinforced by the fact that the patient has no chest or abdominal pain on questioning.

What interventions should be considered for the patient's acute injuries?
- The patient's arms should be placed in a splint or sling, depending on local protocols and the patient's position of comfort.
- If the breath sounds are bilaterally equal and the patient has no chest or abdominal pain, then little else needs to be done in the acute phase for the bruises on the abdomen and chest.

How can the history be clarified?
- One approach is for you and your partner to separate, with one of you talking to the son and the other talking to the patient. This may increase the chances of the patient speaking out and giving better information on what is going on.
- Another strategy is to ask the father and the son for as detailed an explanation as possible. This may expose vagueness in the history and inconsistencies between the stories of the father and the son.

What are your initial management and treatment priorities?
- BLS treatment priorities:
  1. Obtain a detailed history.
  2. Monitor the patient for any deterioration.
  3. Splint the extremity.
  4. Provide an outlet for the patient to talk if they wish.
  5. Transport in position of comfort.

Note to instructor: Discuss the following only if you are using this scenario with an ALS audience. Skip this part when discussing with a BLS audience.
- ALS treatment priorities:
  1. BLS priorities, plus provide any advanced intervention as dictated by the patient's situation.
  2. Consider intravenous access while en route to the emergency department; this may be useful for analgesia both in the prehospital and in the emergency department setting.

■ Issues in Management

- The issue of managing the right arm injury is straightforward: it should be splinted and/or placed in a sling as indicated.
- Given the fact that the bruises involve the chest and the abdomen, the patient should be observed for signs of any other injuries. Otherwise, these contusions do not have relevance to acute trauma.
- Perhaps the most important issue in management is to attempt to reconcile vagueness and inconsistencies between the stories of father and son and in terms of the multiple signs of injury on the patient.

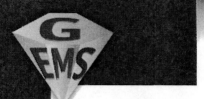

Section 3: Scenarios

■ Case Development

The patient's situation remains unchanged during the transport; he says very little during transport and the son does all the talking. It turns out that the son lives with his father, and the son pays a nominal rent to the father for the living quarters. The son has a history of alcoholism and is on disability for this; therefore he is in part financially dependent on the father. Upon arrival at the receiving institution, the son continues to give a vague history of causes of the father's bruises, stating, "My father falls a lot." At first the father has little to add to this, but when he is questioned separately from the son with direct questioning, he states that his son has struck him in anger. The father is afraid his son will "get into trouble" and he does not want that to occur.

■ Core Knowledge Points

What are risk factors for abuse of the older person?
- Older persons who have some dementia or other cognitive impairment are at particular risk for abuse. These patients may not be believed if they talk about abuse.
- The abuse victim may have poor health and functional impairment, and thus be particularly vulnerable.
- There is frequently a dependence of the abusing party on the abuse victim. In this case, the son is partially financially dependent on the father.
- The abuser may have a history of violence, but this may be difficult to ascertain in the prehospital setting.
- The abuser and abuse victim often have a shared living arrangement.

What presentations suggest abuse of an older patient?
- Similar to pediatric abuse, the following may be seen:
  1. Delays between an injury or illness and seeking medical attention
  2. Disparity in histories from the patient and the suspected abuser
  3. Implausible or vague explanations provided by either party
  4. Frequent visits to the emergency room

What questions may identify possible abuse?
- Sometimes direct questioning is the best approach. A simple question "Has anyone at home hurt you?" may give the answer.
- When direct questioning fails, sometimes indirect questioning may provide important information. An example of indirect questioning is "Are you receiving enough care at home?"

What should you do if abuse is suspected?
- Report inconsistencies in the story, vagueness from family members describing patient injuries, or other suspicious incidents to the receiving hospital.
- Suspected elder abuse may be a reportable event, just as for pediatric abuse; follow local protocols for reporting.
- The National Center of Elder Abuse is a resource for further information on this topic:

National Center on Elder Abuse
1225 I Street, NW, Suite 725
Washington, D.C. 20005

■ Summary

This patient did not have a serious injury, but the patient's situation was serious. Multiple injures, vague stories, unwillingness to be straightforward with the history—these are a few of the potential warnings for an elder abuse situation. Because you actually witness the patient's living situation, you are more likely to be able to see the clues to elder abuse. Always report suspicions of abuse or neglect to the receiving hospital and to appropriate authorities as dictated by your local protocols.

Section 3: Scenarios

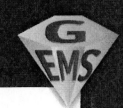

BLS Scenarios: Delirium vs. Dementia

This case is designed to facilitate discussion on delirium and dementia. The patient is stable with a recent history of gradual changes in her mental status (multi-infarct dementia). Discussion should be centered on the importance of differentiating delirium from dementia.

■ Objectives

At the completion of this scenario, the student will be able to:
- Discuss the definition of delirium and dementia.
- Distinguish between delirium and dementia.
- Formulate a plan to evaluate the older patient with a complaint related to delirium or dementia.

■ Case Presentation

You are dispatched to the home of a 70-year-old woman who has been reported by family members as "acting strangely." When they called 9-1-1, the family members reported that over the past few months, the patient has had difficulty remembering people and places that she normally would have known. They also report a decrease in the patient's functional ability to handle activities of daily living like getting dressed or brushing her hair. Although the patient can still talk, the family noted decreased language skills. The patient's son and daughter, who are present and who called 9-1-1, state that the patient's decline has been gradual over the past few months, but during this weekly visit they noticed a functional decline that they are concerned is making the patient unable to care for herself. They say that the patient has hypertension, for which she takes an unknown medication, and a history of "strokes" for which she takes a "blood thinner." No other information is attainable from the family at this time.

■ Faculty Information

Initial Assessment
ABCDEs:
- Airway: The airway is open and there are no signs of obstruction.
- Breathing: The patient is breathing at 16 breaths/min with excellent bilateral breath sounds and oxygen saturation of 100%.
- Circulation: The heart rate is 72 beats/min with a blood pressure of 120/80 mm Hg.
- Disability: The patient is alert and conversant. The patient knows her name but is incorrect when asked the date or her mailing address. She states she is "having trouble remembering" these things.
- Exposure: There are no signs of trauma on inspection of the patient.

SAMPLE History:
- Signs: Per the son, a decreasing level of orientation.
- Allergies: No known allergies
- Medications: Unknown antihypertensive and blood thinner
- Past history: Hypertension, CVA
- Last meal: Breakfast 3 hours ago
- Events leading up: Gradual decreasing of orientation

ALS Information:
- ECG: Normal sinus rhythm without ectopy
- Blood sugar: 140 mg/dL
- Temperature: 98.8°F

♦ GEMS diamond:
- G: Patient has had difficulty remembering over last few months, decrease in functional ability (ADLs), decreased language skills. Greater decline today.
- E: Nothing noted.
- M: Patient is taking a blood thinner and an unknown medication for hypertension.
- S: Daughter and son are present and appear concerned.

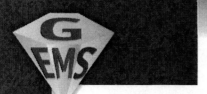

Section 3: Scenarios

The patient has no evidence of trauma or acute hemodynamic compromise, but there is evidence of a gradually worsening mental status with functional deterioration over two months.

Management Strategies

Based on this patient's presentation, what are likely causes of the patient's altered mental status?
- One possibility is that the patient has multi-infarct dementia. This is made more likely by the fact that the patient has had strokes in the past. Multi-infarct dementia, caused by multiple small strokes, can present with an apparent gradual decline.
- Alzheimer's-type dementia is another possibility. Alzheimer's is characterized by a gradual onset and continuing decline and has deficits which are relatively constant over the course of a day.
- There may also be a metabolic or toxic explanation for the gradual decline. For example, the patient could have a hyponatremia syndrome, which can have neurological manifestations. The patient could also have thyroid disease or some drug toxicity.
- Trauma is also a possibility, as older patients are relatively likely to sustain falls and may not report these falls due to either minimizing their importance or being afraid to have family members think they may need to be institutionalized. The patient's blood thinner medication will not make her more likely to fall, but she is predisposed to hematoma formation when she does fall.

What is the patient's physiologic status?
- The patient is hemodynamically stable with no acute neurologic crisis present.
- Keep in mind the VITAMINS C&D mnemonic when considering potential causes:
    - V *Vascular*: stroke, brain embolism
    - I *Inflammation*: inflammation of the blood vessels in the brain (vasculitis)
    - T *Toxins*: carbon monoxide poisoning
       Trauma: concussion, intracerebral hemorrhage
       Tumors: primary brain tumor or tumor that developed elsewhere and spread to the brain (metastasis)
    - A *Autoimmune*: production of immune system components against a normal structure in the central nervous system
    - M *Metabolic*: liver or renal failure, hypoglycemia, hyperglycemia, hypothyroidism, nonketotic diabetic acidosis
    - I *Infection*: meningitis, encephalitis
    - N *Narcotics or other drugs*: many possibilities, with a higher chance of mental status changes if there is pre-existing brain disease.
    - S *Systemic*: sepsis, hypoxia
    - C *Congenital*: seizures
    - D *Degenerative*: Alzheimer's disease and other dementias, Parkinson's disease

What are the initial management and treatment priorities?
- BLS treatment priorities:
    1. As stabilization and transport continue, obtain a more complete history.
    2. Maintain the airway and monitor blood pressure during evaluation and transport.
    3. Obtain more history from family members and encourage them to accompany the patient to the hospital where a more detailed history can be given.

Note to instructor: Discuss the following only if you are using this scenario with an ALS audience. Skip this part when discussing with a BLS audience.
- ALS treatment priorities:
    1. BLS priorities, plus monitor for the need for advanced airway, breathing, or circulation support maneuvers.
    2. Attempt intravenous access on the way to the emergency department.

Section 3: Scenarios

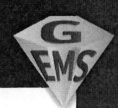

Issues in Management
- This patient's vital signs are stable and she does not have any acute neurologic crisis. Your priorities, therefore, are to get a useful history, stabilize and transport the patient to the emergency department, and take whatever steps can be taken to maximize the chances of appropriate diagnosis at the receiving hospital. Along these lines, you should assess medication lists, any unusual events occurring in the time period surrounding the patient's onset of mental decline, and any other potentially pertinent aspects of the history.

Core Knowledge Points

What are the characteristics of dementia in the older population?
- Dementia is defined as an acquired decline in memory and also in at least one other cognitive function (such as language or the ability to perform activities of daily living) sufficient to effect daily life in an alert person.
- The causes of dementia in the older population include Alzheimer's dementia, which is the most frequent cause, and other progressive disorders such as multi-infarct dementia. There are other, reversible, causes of dementia which include drug toxicity and metabolic as well as neurologic (hematoma, normal pressure hydrocephalus) explanations.

How are the multiple potential causes of dementia distinguished?
- Alzheimer's dementia is characterized by a gradual onset with continuing decline and the absence of other explanations for the dementia. Alzheimer's patients may have some manifestations of delirium, but deficits also occur in the absence of delirium.
- Patients may have altered mental status due to drug toxicities; your primary contribution in this area is to get a complete drug listing and bring medications to the hospital.
- Metabolic changes can also be responsible for apparent dementia. Be sure to obtain as complete a medical history as possible.
- Thyroid disease may also cause dementia; take a thorough past medical history and note any surgical scars on the neck that may indicate previous surgery.
- In patients with a history of head trauma, traumatic brain injury is the likely cause of dementia.

Case Development
This older woman had a gradual onset of dementia-like symptoms which progressed over a period of a couple of months, to the point where family members called 9-1-1. On further questioning, the family members reported that their mother was a "minimizer" of symptoms who rarely communicates with her family about any medical symptoms she may have. The family expressed concerns that the patient has had strokes in the past and may have some problems with balance. They stated that the patient has been evasive when asked if she had fallen. Based on this history, the EMS providers expressed to the receiving facility their concerns that this patient may have a history of falling and a possible chronic hematoma. Imaging at the hospital confirmed this suspicion, and the patient subsequently underwent a successful treatment and recovery.

Summary
Dementia should be considered a diagnosis of exclusion. Older patients with altered mental status are frequently encountered; you should have a high index of suspicion for non-dementia causes of altered mental status. To determine the cause, tests may need to be conducted at the hospital. In many cases, the history provided by EMS can help focus the emergency department evaluator's attention appropriately for alternative causes of "dementia."

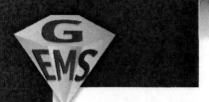

Section 3: Scenarios

ALS Scenarios: Communication Challenges

The scenarios portion of the concurrent skill/scenario station on Communication and Assessment is 45 minutes long and designed to cover two scenarios. When you are finished discussing this scenario, move on to the BLS communication scenario on page 149.

These scenarios are applicable to both BLS and ALS audiences. This case is designed to facilitate discussion on the importance of communication with the older patient. The patient is stable with a recent history of a clinically significant syncopal episode and would like to refuse care. Discussion should be centered on communication with the older patient, however, clinical aspects of the syncope are also discussed.

▪ Objectives

At the completion of this scenario, the student will be able to:
- Analyze the needs of an older patient with sensory deficits.
- Formulate a plan to better communicate with an older patient with sensory deficits.

▪ Case Presentation

You are a paramedic dispatched to the home of an 81-year-old woman who had a witnessed syncopal event in her home. While her daughter was visiting, she saw her mother suddenly lose her balance and fall to the floor while walking from the table to the sink. The fall did not appear to induce significant trauma. The patient does not recall what happened, but the daughter reports that the patient was unconscious for 5 to 10 seconds. Upon regaining consciousness (according to the daughter), the patient stated that this sort of thing had happened once or twice a week over the last month or so but that she did not think that it was a significant problem and had not mentioned it to her physician. She had not seen her physician for six months due to missing the last two appointments.

The daughter was concerned enough about the fainting spell to call EMS, but she reports that her mother was angry when she found out that her daughter called EMS. When you arrive at the scene, the patient says, "I feel fine. I don't need to go to the hospital." The patient has no complaints, denies any symptoms, and reiterates her opinion that she does not need to go to the hospital. The daughter, however, is upset at the prospect of her mother not wanting to seek medical attention, and asks you for your assistance in convincing the patient that medical assessment is necessary.

▪ Faculty Information

Initial Assessment
ABCDEs:
- Airway: Open, no signs of obstruction
- Breathing: Respiratory rate is 14 breaths/min and there are good bilateral breath sounds; your initial oxygen saturation reading is 96%.
- Circulation: The heart rate is 72 beats/min, skin is warm and well perfused, and blood pressure is 140/88 mmHg.
- Disability: The patient is alert and has spontaneous eye opening and has no apparent neurologic abnormalities.
- Exposure: There are no signs of injury, contusion, or bony abnormality on inspection of the patient.

ALS Information:
- ECG: 1st degree atrioventricular block
- Blood sugar: 134 mg/dL

SAMPLE History:
- Signs: Per the daughter, the patient fainted.
- Allergies: Penicillin
- Medications: Cardizem, Nitro-Dur patch

Section 3: Scenarios

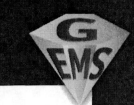

- Past history: Hypertension
- Last meal: Breakfast 2 hours ago
- Events leading up: The daughter states the patient was acting fine this morning.

GEMS diamond:
- G: Patient reports fainting once or twice a week over last month.
- E: Nothing noted.
- M: Patient takes Cardizem, has a Nitro-Dur patch.
- S: Daughter was visiting. Patient does not want to go to hospital and has missed recent doctor appointments.

The patient has evidence of potentially significant syncope, with no signs of trauma resulting from the fall.

■ Management Strategies

Based on this patient's presentation, what are the likely causes of syncope?
- Cardiac
- Neurologic
- Volume depletion
- Medication-related

What is the patient's physiologic status?
- The patient has normal vital signs and no signs of an acute medical or traumatic problem.

What are your initial management (treatment) priorities?
- **BLS treatment priorities:**
  1. As stabilization and initial preparations for transport continue, obtain a more complete history from the patient and the daughter.
  2. Monitor and maintain the airway.
  3. Monitor vital signs.
  4. Monitor for the appearance of new symptoms.
  5. Address the importance of this patient undergoing medical evaluation for syncope, and also to search for other injuries related to her fall (or previous falls that may have gone unreported because they were not witnessed).

- **ALS treatment priorities:**
  1. BLS priorities, plus advanced airway or hemodynamic support if the patient deteriorates.
  2. Attempt intravenous access.
  3. Check blood sugar and administer dextrose if indicated.
  4. A 12-lead ECG should be attempted if time permits.

■ Issues in Management

- This patient had a syncopal episode which obviously warrants further evaluation and probable hospitalization, but she initially insists that she is "fine, and doesn't need transport to the hospital." In fact, the patient is hemodynamically stable, has no clear ongoing neurologic problems, and other than the treatment priorities as noted above, does not actually require much in the way of urgent medical intervention.
- The primary management issue in this case is more related to psychological evaluation and support skills than to medical interventions. Remember that psychological and emotional support are critical in emergency treatment of older patients. Specifically, this patient seems insistent that she does not want to go to the hospital for evaluation. EMS providers could, very strictly speaking, judge her to be mentally competent and not in need of emergency medical intervention, and have her sign a "refusal for transport" form and decline hospital evaluation. However, such an approach is clearly not in the best interests of the patient. Of all the cutting-edge interventions which can be provided for patients with syncope, none are useful if they can't be implemented because of a patient's refusal

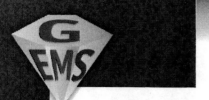

Section 3: Scenarios

of transport. The critical issue in this case is to explore the reasons for the patient's reticence for hospital evaluation see if these reasons can be addressed, and make the patient comfortable with the knowledge that hospitalization is both indicated and potentially useful.

Core Knowledge Points

When do patients with syncope need to be evaluated in the hospital?
- Medical evaluation of syncope is not the main issue in this scenario, but you should have familiarity with disease processes so that you can give reasonable and relevant advice to patients, especially those who wish to refuse transport. For the older population, any patient who has syncope should be transported to the hospital for further evaluation. There is a relatively high risk of a serious cause for the fainting spell. Providers who are aware of this can more rationally discuss the need for transport with a reluctant patient.

What should you do when a patient wishes to refuse transport?
- First of all, try to understand the patient's rationale for refusing transport. If a patient has an errant reasoning behind not wishing to be transported, and this reasoning can be easily shown to be faulty, patients will often change their mind and consent to transport. This is preferable to transporting patients against their will, even when the latter is technically appropriate. If patients are clearly not within their mental faculties, then the initial attempt to expose their faulty reasoning should be short, but it is still worth the time.
- Patients who do not require emergency medical treatment and who seem to have intact judgment—and thus can "legally" refuse transport—provide a challenge to EMS providers. In such a case, the patient cannot and should not be transported against his or her will, but you do have some tools to use in your attempts to get the patient to consent to transport. The first tool is the family member, who is at hand and is presumably trusted by the patient. Explain the reasons for transport to the family member while the patient is listening. Sometimes the family member can then help the patient understand the need for transport. The family member can also help discuss the patient's concerns regarding transport. In short, while in some cases patients must be transported against their will, it is always preferable to have discussions with the patient (and family when present) so that by the time the transport commences, all interested parties are in agreement that it is the right thing to do. Simply having the patient sign a transport refusal form, or alternatively simply performing a quick assessment followed by bundling of the patient into the ambulance against his or her will, are not desirable approaches.

How can you "talk patients into being transported?"
- Here, the primary advantages that EMS providers have are access to information that patients and families may not have about disease processes, and a perceived objective viewpoint. While in some cases patients refusing transport may require specialized psychiatric services, most of the time simply discussing the facts with the patient and getting to the bottom of their reluctance to be transported will lead to a good outcome.

Case Development

As you discuss the case with the patient and her daughter, explaining why it is important for patients with syncope to be evaluated at the hospital, the patient begins to open up and explain her reluctance to be transported. It turns out that the patient has had two friends, in approximately her age range, who have been transported to the hospital with various complaints within the past two months; neither one of these acquaintances ever left the hospital as one died and the other ended up requiring nursing home placement. The patient has an understandable level of anxiety about being transported to the hospital, because

Section 3: Scenarios

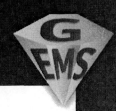

transport to the hospital has been something of a one-way trip for her two friends. Armed with the understanding of the patient's concerns, you can then explain that even when syncope has a serious cause, these are often quite amenable to treatment. Also explain that the evaluation and treatment of syncope are much more likely to result in a good outcome than if the patient stays at home and continues to have the episodes. In this case, the patient then consented to transfer to the hospital and the remainder of the transport was uneventful.

■ Summary

Sometimes it is psychological, rather than medical, support and intervention that is most important. In a case like this, when a patient does not require emergency intervention but definitely requires hospital evaluation and management, the most important thing EMS providers can do is to convince the patient to go to the hospital where these interventions can occur. Many times, older patients will have had friends or family go to the hospital for seemingly minor problems, only to not return. Older patients' anxiety over such a one-way trip to the hospital is quite understandable. This anxiety is best addressed with knowledge, objectivity, and reassurance.

- When patients refuse transport to the hospital, try to talk with them and explain the reason transport is needed.
- Family members should be involved in these conversations with the patient whenever possible, so the patient can benefit both from your objective viewpoint and the advice of loved ones. (However, in some cases, the presence of family members may not be helpful, and patients may in fact feel that people are "ganging up on them." Use your judgment when determining whether conversations with a patient should involve family. Avoid giving an older patient the impression that they are being ignored in the decision-making process. This impression is all too easily given when EMS providers discuss the case with the patient's family members and do not involve the patient.
- While you should never create transport delays that endanger the patient, it is always better to transport a patient willingly rather than against his or her will. Consider taking time to talk with the patient when possible. This is time well spent.
- When a patient who has reasonable judgment and competence refuses transport, the seemingly quickest "solution" of having them sign a transport refusal form is very frequently not in the best interest of the patient. Investigate the patient's reasoning, and try to do what is best for the patient.

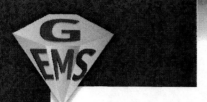

Section 3: Scenarios

ALS Scenarios: Do Not Resuscitate Orders

Note to Faculty: Because of differences in local protocols, this scenario requires some customization. Before the course, prepare samples of valid DNR orders to show students, and also bring documents that are not valid per your local protocol if possible.

This case is designed to facilitate discussion on do not resuscitate (DNR) orders. The patient is unstable but requires initial care, before becoming pulseless and apneic. Discussion should include local protocols regarding DNR orders and what must be done to honor them. Advance directives should also be discussed.

Objectives

At the completion of this scenario, the student will be able to:
- Recognize a valid DNR order in their local jurisdiction.
- Identify the wishes of a patient with a DNR order.
- Explain the psychological impact of sudden stressors on both family and EMS providers.

Case Presentation

You are dispatched to a nursing home for an 84-year-old man who is having severe chest pain. By the time you arrive at the patient's side, he has lost consciousness and has a bradycardic rhythm with a faintly palpable carotid pulse. You apply oxygen and you and your partner begin your assessment of the patient. The nursing home floor nurse supervisor presents to you a DNR document that is valid in your jurisdiction for the patient in question.

Faculty Information

Initial Assessment

ABCDEs:
- Airway: Snoring, erratic respirations
- Breathing: Respiratory rate is 10 breaths/min and there are diminished breath sounds; your initial oxygen saturation reading is 82%.
- Circulation: Heart rate is 36 beats/min; ECG shows sinus bradycardia with frequent multifocal premature ventricular contractions (PVCs); skin is cool, pale, mottled, cyanotic around lips/fingernails.
- Disability: The patient is unresponsive.
- Exposure: There are no signs of trauma.

GEMS diamond:
- G: Nursing home patient with severe chest pain.
- E: Nothing noted.
- M: None noted.
- S: Nursing home staff presents valid DNR document.

Initial assessment showed a patient who clearly needed both airway management and ACLS protocol-guided cardiac therapy. Before any interventions could be provided, a valid DNR order was presented. During initial assessment and treatment, the patient's ECG changes to ventricular fibrillation and the patient becomes pulseless.

Management Strategies

Note to Faculty: At this point, hold a discussion regarding the local protocol regarding DNR in your area. Show the samples of valid DNR orders and documents that are not valid per your local protocol. Have students review the forms and assess whether or not they are valid.

Should this patient undergo resuscitation?
- The patient is in cardiorespiratory arrest and, if there were no DNR order, would require intervention.
- The patient has a valid DNR order document presented to EMS. (For jurisdictions where this is applicable, it should also be assumed that the patient is wearing the appropriate "DNR bracelet.")

Section 3: Scenarios

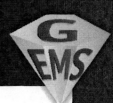

Since the patient has a DNR order in force, the management strategies for this particular scenario revolve around "non-medical" issues.
- ALS and BLS treatment priorities are similar.
- Though no medical treatment is indicated, there are interventions and interactions which are appropriate for EMS providers at a scene such as this.

Issues in Management

- Unfortunately, it is not uncommon for EMS providers to be called to a patient who has a DNR order in force, but who otherwise requires cardiopulmonary resuscitation. In this particular instance, EMS had been called while the patient still had a perfusing pulse and a clinical picture consistent with acute myocardial infarction. It is of primary importance to note that a DNR order does not mean that patients should not receive appropriate medical therapy up to the interventions that are precluded by the DNR order. A patient with the DNR order who has severe chest pain should be treated for that chest pain. Therefore, in this case it was completely appropriate for EMS to be called to the patient. In some other cases, however, EMS may be called when the medical indications are not so clear. For example, a terminal cancer patient who dies at home may prompt a call to the EMS service. An important issue for EMS providers in interacting with family members or caregivers is to be sympathetic to the difficult situation in which family members find themselves witnessing the death of a loved one. Remember that while you have probably seen patients die before, most individuals have not, precipitating a call to EMS.
- Interpersonal interactions are paramount in the evaluation of a DNR patient. First of all, it is only with skilled interpersonal relations that a DNR order can be rapidly produced and evaluated by EMS providers. Once this is determined to be in force, discuss the reasoning behind non-resuscitation decision-making with any family members present. Of course, patients should always be made comfortable and provided appropriate medical therapy if they still have a perfusing pulse and respirations.
- It is very difficult for EMS providers to "stand by and do nothing" even though a valid DNR often mandates just such a course. It is normal to feel uncomfortable watching a patient die, when all your instincts are to intervene. If this stress becomes overwhelming, this should become a part of critical incident stress management.
- DNR situations can occur in the patient's home. Do not simply note that the DNR is in force, state that the patient has died, and leave. Instead, provide empathic care for family members, helping with appropriate logistics (eg, death notification).
- It is always a good idea to discuss the situation with family members. Whether the issue is the meaning of the DNR order, difficulty of "standing by and doing nothing," or helping the family contact a funeral home, the more communication and psychological assistance you can provide the better.

Note to Faculty: Local protocols should be discussed during this scenario. If available, show local forms, bracelets or other documentation to students for review. Local protocols regarding advance directives, living wills, durable power of attorney, or health care proxies should also be discussed here.

Summary

DNR situations are highly region-specific, and the individual approach of an EMS provider is quite dependent on the laws and protocols in the region. However, some common sense rules apply universally. Concentrate on quickly validating any possible DNR orders, determining which therapies are and are not precluded by these orders, and then act in line with the patient's expressed wishes as per the DNR order.

Communication with patient family members and caregivers is an important part of managing the scene in cases like this. As an EMS provider, you are well positioned to provide sympathetic care to the family.

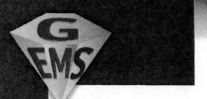

Section 3: Scenarios

ALS Scenarios: Stroke

This case is designed to facilitate discussion on care of the older patient with a CVA. The patient is unstable with a recent history of a hemorrhagic stroke. Discussion should be centered on the management and transport of the older patient who has experienced a stroke.

▪ Objectives

At the completion of this scenario, the student will be able to:
- Recognize the signs and symptoms of an older patient experiencing a possible stroke.
- Determine the proper treatment for an older patient experiencing a possible stroke.
- Recall the need to determine the time of onset of symptoms when completing the patient history.

▪ Case Presentation

Your service is dispatched to the home of an 80-year-old man who complained of a sudden onset of a severe headache and then fell to the floor. Family members who are present noted that the patient has been unconscious since the incident, which was 20 minutes prior to your arrival, and the patient is in that status upon your arrival.

▪ Faculty Information

Initial Assessment
ABCDEs:
- Airway: The patient's airway is partially blocked by his tongue, which has prolapsed posteriorly and is producing snoring sounds.
- Breathing: The respiratory rate is 6 to 8 breaths/min, and the breaths are shallow and irregular with limited chest rise.
- Circulation: His blood pressure is 240/160 mmHg and the heart rate is 56 beats/min. The skin is pale, warm and dry, and distal pulses are present.
- Disability: The patient has a withdrawal response to pain but does not move his extremities spontaneously, has no spontaneous eye opening, and is nonverbal.
- Exposure: There are no signs of trauma to the patient's head or the remainder of his body.

SAMPLE History:
- Signs: Patient is responsive only to pain with decerebrate posturing.
- Allergies: Denied by the son.
- Medications: Vasotec, Lopressor, and hydrochlothiazide, but the patient often forgets to take his medications.
- Past history: The son tells you that the patient has a long-standing history of poorly controlled hypertension but has no other past medical history.
- Last meal: Breakfast 2 hours earlier
- Events leading up: The patient's son, who called the ambulance, tells you that the patient complained of a sudden onset of a very severe headache, followed by loss of consciousness within seconds and an apparently comatose state, in which he remains.

ALS Information:
- ECG: Sinus bradycardia
- Blood sugar: 140 mg/dL
- Pulse Ox: 86% on room air

Section 3: Scenarios

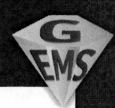

- GEMS diamond:
  - G: Patient had sudden severe headache, fell to floor. History of poorly controlled hypertension.
  - E: Nothing noted.
  - M: Patient often forgets to take his Vasotec, Lasopressor, and hydrochlorthiazide.
  - S: Family members are present.

For this patient, with a history of hypertension and a clinical picture suggestive of an acute neurologic event, stroke is the most likely diagnosis.

Management Strategies

What are the initial management priorities for this patient?
- The patient needs to have emergency airway support and definitive intervention.
- Depending on local protocols, the patient may need to have his blood pressure controlled by an agent which decreases the pressure.

What is the patient's neurologic status?
- The patient is minimally responsive. He is unable to give any history and needs airway intervention. He is, however, withdrawing to pain, giving him a Glasgow Coma Scale Score of 6 (eye opening = 1, motor = 4, verbal = 1).

Issues in Management

- The simple intervention of ensuring oxygenation is vital in this patient, since hypoxemia can contribute to neurologic injury.
- No signs of volume depletion are present, and volume overloading can cause injury in patients with an acute neurologic event. The patient does need IV access, but overzealous fluid administration should be avoided.
- The patient's hypertension and bradycardia may represent a Cushing's response, which could be indicative of an impending herniation. Overzealous lowering of the blood pressure can blunt the ability of this response to maintain intracranial perfusion pressure. Blood pressure should be managed in conjunction with local protocols and/or contact with medical control.
- The history of the current event and past medical history should be confirmed, since it is unlikely that the patient will be able to provide this (or other) information at the receiving hospital.
- Initial and ongoing assessment of neurologic status is very important, since this status can change frequently and may in fact deteriorate while providers are en route to the receiving hospital.

Case Development

The patient's situation deteriorates during the transport, such that his Glasgow Coma Scale score becomes 3. Intubation is performed early in his transport and the hemodynamic parameters are addressed with peri-intubation benzodiazepines in the field, with specific anti-hypertensives administered upon hospital arrival. A CT scan done soon after arrival shows a large subarachnoid and intraparenchymal hemorrhage with some midline shift and signs of early herniation.

Core Knowledge Points

Differences in history point to hemorrhagic versus nonhemorrhagic stroke.
- Probably the most important finding, as was present in this patient, is the fact that a severe sudden headache occurred. This is much more likely to be present in the case of a hemorrhagic stroke than in a nonhemorrhagic stroke.
- The history of long-standing hypertension also suggests a hemorrhagic stroke. Recent history of head trauma or fall may also indicate a hemorrhagic stroke.

Section 3: Scenarios

Supportive therapies should be provided for patients with hemorrhagic and nonhemorrhagic stroke.
- The airway should be supported, with early intubation provided as indicated. A single oxygen desaturation below 90% risks worsened neurologic outcome.
- Hemodynamic support for the patient is limited in order to avoid fluid overload, and blood pressure is carefully monitored. Some EMS systems may allow for acute blood pressure management in the field, but this is usually left to the hospital setting. Blood pressure management in the case of acute stroke is an evolving field. In general, the systolic blood pressure should not be lowered if it is less than 180 mm Hg. Even if the blood pressure is high (above 180 to 200 mm Hg), it should be lowered only gently.
- Euglycemia is important in acute stroke. Hypoglycemia can masquerade as just about any neurologic syndrome and it should be sought and treated as indicated. On the other hand, hyperglycemia is known to cause injury in the case of an acute neurologic event; thus administration of dextrose-containing fluids is not recommended for stroke patients.

What is the role of hyperventilation management in acute stroke?
- Hyperventilation management is a temporizing therapy which should be employed in patients only as a "bridge" to more definitive therapy (such as neurosurgery).
- Overzealous hyperventilation contributes to a worsened outcome, and thus hyperventilation therapy is not recommended in the prehospital setting unless there are signs of active herniation.

What are the signs of herniation?
- Signs of herniation include profound decerebrate posturing, a single "blown pupil," and for patients who have a Glasgow Coma Scale score of less than 9, an acute decrease of 2 points in their score.

What are the prehospital definitive treatments for hemorrhagic stroke?
- There are no definitive treatments for stroke in the prehospital setting. Supportive measures (eg, oxygen, blood pressure support) can be very important. Hyperventilation is rarely appropriate, but may be required. In some cases mannitol may be used (depending on local protocols) when signs of herniation are present.
- Even though specific interventions are usually not provided in the prehospital setting, there is mounting evidence that close attention to supportive care (such as airway management) improves the outcome for these patients.

Summary

Acute ischemic stroke has received much attention in the literature lately, and the prehospital field is a fertile area of research and clinical change in the care of these patients. Unfortunately, patients with hemorrhagic stroke continue to have a high acuity and a poor outcome. Rapid response, aggressive supportive care, and adequate and succinct history are priorities for these patients. Reporting this and the physical findings to the receiving hospital can help expedite care of these critical patients and improve outcome when this is possible.

Section 3: Scenarios

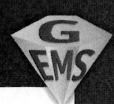

ALS Scenarios: Medication Interactions

This case is designed to facilitate discussion on the importance of medication history and common medication problems. The patient is unstable with a recent history of a clinically significant syncopal episode from a medication error. Discussion should be centered on the clinical aspects of the syncope and the importance of obtaining a complete medication history.

■ Objectives

At the completion of this scenario, the student will be able to:
- Determine the need to obtain a complete medication history for the older patient.
- Specify the components of a complete medication history.
- Formulate a plan to evaluate the older patient with a complaint related to a medication reaction.

■ Case Presentation

Your ALS unit is dispatched to the home of an 82-year-old woman who has been witnessed to have a syncopal event while seated at dinner. The patient did not fall and there is no history of trauma. The patient was eating with three other acquaintances and complained of feeling weak, then slumped over. The patient is still unconscious upon your arrival at the scene. The patient has no family members who are currently available to help with the history, and the acquaintances dining with the patient do not know her past medical history.

■ Faculty Information

Initial Assessment
ABCDEs:
- Airway: The airway is currently open. There are no signs of acute obstruction.
- Breathing: The respiratory rate is 16 breaths/min and there are good bilateral breath sounds with appropriate chest rise; oxygen saturation is 97%.
- Circulation: The heart rate is difficult to determine by palpating the pulse, as the radial pulse is faint. No blood pressure is obtainable using a brachial (arm) cuff. The patient seems to have a very faint femoral pulse as well; the femoral pulse rate of approximately 20 to 30 beats/min is confirmed by palpation of the carotid pulse.
- Disability: The patient is responsive only to painful stimulus, and localizes pain appropriately. There is no spontaneous eye opening and the patient does not open the eyes in response to verbal stimulus.
- Exposure: There are no signs of trauma upon inspection of the patient.

SAMPLE History:
- Signs: Unresponsive
- Allergies: Unknown
- Medications: Unknown
- Past history: Unknown
- Last meal: She was eating dinner at the time of the incident
- Events leading up: The patient felt weak then passed out.

ALS Information:
- ECG: Junctional rhythm
- Blood sugar: 440 mg/dL
- 12-lead ECG: Junctional rhythm with high grade AV block
- GEMS diamond:
  - G: While eating dinner, patient complained of feeling weak, then fainted.
  - E: Nothing noted.
  - M: Unknown
  - S: Patient was eating with three acquaintances, has no family available to give history.

Section 3: Scenarios

This patient has evidence of significant hemodynamic compromise, with both bradycardia and hypotension.

Management Strategies

Based on this patient's presentation, what are the treatment priorities?
- The airway is open at this point, but the patient has significant neurologic compromise and consideration should be given to intubating the patient for airway protection.
- The primary problem with this patient is hemodynamic collapse as evidenced by bradycardia and hypotension. A management priority is establishment of adequate intravenous access with administration of intravenous fluids and/or agents for blood pressure support.
- After the patient has been stabilized during preparations for transport, a very brief history should be sought from those who were dining with the patient or other sources of information, in an attempt to determine possible explanations for the patient's presentation. Though transport should not be unduly delayed to obtain this information, it is important to take a minute or two to try and obtain information as you are in the best position to get any pertinent data.

Based on the patient's presentation, what are the likely causes of the syncope?
- Since the patient was eating during the episode, a foreign body (aspiration) is a possible cause of syncope. This seems unlikely since the patient's airway and breathing were okay on initial evaluation.
- An acute coronary syndrome can always be responsible for syncope, especially if there is associated bradycardia and/or hypotension.
- An acute cerebrovascular event may also explain a syncopal episode. The information given in the case thus far is insufficient to allow you to rule out a neurologic explanation for the patient's presentation; however, there is little specific therapy which would be indicated in the setting of a neurologic explanation, so you do not need to focus further on this possibility at this point.
- An additional explanation for the patient's syncope could be a metabolic abnormality, or a toxicologic or medication-related problem. This represents a wide array of possible diagnoses, and further focusing of the medical history would be necessary to identify likely explanations along these lines.

What are the BLS and ALS initial treatment priorities and management options at this point?
- BLS treatment priorities:
    1. Move the patient from a sitting position in the chair to flat on the floor.
    2. Maintain the patient's airway and monitor blood pressure.
    3. Provide rapid transport and/or assist ALS providers, especially with obtaining history while the ALS providers (if present) provide advanced medical stabilization.
    4. Monitor the appearance of any new symptoms or any changes in status.

- ALS treatment priorities:
    1. BLS priorities, plus consider intubation if the patient does not appear to be able to protect the airway.
    2. Intravenous access is critical in this patient, who has hemodynamic compromise.
    3. Fluid resuscitation and potential contact with medical control for pharmacologic measures to treat the patient's bradycardia and hypotension.
    4. Provide any treatment indicated by initial evaluation (for example, if the rapid reagent glucose check is low, dextrose administration; administration of naloxone if there are pinpoint pupils).
    5. Ongoing ECG monitoring with 12-lead ECG if available.

Section 3: Scenarios

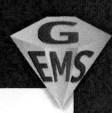

■ Issues in Management
- The patient is hemodynamically unstable, with significant bradycardia as well as hypotension. Other than the fact that the pulse is palpable in the femoral area, there is no specific blood pressure noted. Continue to monitor the pulse and evaluate blood pressure by traditional means when this is possible. Notably, the patient should not have repeated assessments of the carotid pulse. There are two reasons for this: One is that older patients may be particularly susceptible to bradycardia as a result of carotid stimulation; this would be particularly problematic in this patient who is already manifesting significant bradycardia. Second, repeated carotid palpation is not a good idea in the older population since this group is more likely to have carotid vascular disease. This disease process is associated with risk of iatrogenic embolic stroke from repeated carotid pulse checks (especially if these pulse checks are vigorous, as is likely to occur in the field).
- The patient is breathing and has an acceptable oxygen saturation, but the airway is at risk as long as the profound neurologic compromise continues. Ongoing assessment and decision-making should address whether or not advanced airway maneuvers are necessary.
- As long as the patient has hypotension associated with bradycardia, specific interventions for the bradycardia are indicated. Depending on your local protocol, these may include drug administration (such as atropine) or electrical (external pacemaker) mechanisms. The patient should also receive intravenous fluids for blood pressure support; vasopressor agents may also be necessary.
- Once the airway, breathing, and circulation have been reasonably addressed, the priority is to expedite transport to the hospital setting. Balance this overriding need for rapid stabilization in transport with the fact that in many circumstances, there may be critical aspects to the history which are best (or only) obtained by you at the scene. Other personnel at the scene (such as a BLS unit) may be able to assist you in trying to obtain more historical information. For example, in this case there is a family member who can be contacted for more information.

■ Core Knowledge Points

What is the role of the history in patients with syncope?
- The history is possibly the single most important aspect to determining the cause of syncope. Syncope is very common in older people, and is more likely to be due to serious (cardiac or neurologic) causes as compared to younger patients. Unfortunately, it is very common for patients who have significant syncopal events to be admitted to the hospital only to have a negative work-up and no ultimate clear diagnosis made. Therefore, any historical clues which can be obtained may be critical in determining the cause of syncope. In this particular instance, it will be worth your time to briefly contact the family member to try and learn something of the patient's past medical history.

What are the clues to the cause of syncope in this patient?
- The fact that the patient's airway seems to be patent suggests that there was no aspiration. The fact that the patient has profound bradycardia as a probable explanation of hypotension suggests a cardiac cause for the patient's presentation. If a 12-lead ECG is available at the scene, or if a good quality rhythm strip can be printed at the scene, consider this important information in trying to determine which cardiac issues may be present.

■ Case Development
This 82-year-old woman had syncope with profound bradycardia and hypotension. During initial stabilization, the patient became more responsive, with demonstrated ability to protect the airway. A rhythm strip showed a junctional escape rhythm with what appeared to be a high-grade atrioventricular block. A rapid reagent blood sugar test revealed the patient to have high blood sugar. The rhythm strip also revealed prominent U-waves. The paramedic treating the patient, who had just attended a toxicology refresher course, suspected that the combination of high-grade AV block, hypotension, hyperglycemia, and rhythm strip showing U-waves indicated a possible calcium channel blocker overdose. The paramedic

Section 3: Scenarios

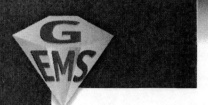

was told by those dining with the patient, in a story which was confirmed by the patient as she recovered her neurologic status, that there was no suicidal intent and that no extra medications had been taken. The daughter was contacted on the telephone and told the providers that the patient's medications were kept in a drawer next to the patient's bed. When the providers got these medications, it was found that the patient was on multiple medications, with at least two different prescribing physicians. One physician, the primary care physician, had prescribed the patient Calan SR, and another physician, a cardiologist, had prescribed the patient Isoptin SR. As the patient recovered enough to answer questions, she confirmed that she was taking both of these medications. The suspicion of calcium channel blocker toxicity was thus confirmed, since these two trade names are both forms of verapamil.

Summary

There may be many explanations for syncope, especially in patients who are initially unable to give a history. Always balance the need for rapid transport with the fact that critical history is best obtained at the scene. In this particular case, the combination of findings prompted EMS to suspect a calcium channel-blocker overdose. The patient may have suffered some deterioration during the transport to the hospital, and thus the information suggesting the true diagnosis could impact patient care (such as selection of a therapeutic intervention with intravenous calcium, glucagon, or a vasopressor).

Additionally, the fact that EMS providers made the connection between multiple medications by multiple prescribing physicians resulted in streamlined patient care at the hospital and helped prevent future problems. Older patients frequently see multiple physicians and there is always the potential for prescriptions interacting or identical medications being unknowingly prescribed by two different physicians. Patients may frequently be unaware of this medication overlap, and if the physicians' offices are geographically separated, prescriptions may be filled at different pharmacies, making it impossible for the pharmacy to catch the error. Overall, this case underlines the critical importance of EMS providers in obtaining a concise yet complete medication history in all older patients.

Section 3: Scenarios

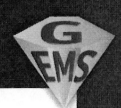

ALS Scenarios: Elder Abuse and Neglect

This case is designed to facilitate discussion on elder abuse and maltreatment. The patient is unstable with an acute onset of worsening shortness of breath, but evidence of neglect is present throughout the assessment. Discussion should be centered on elder abuse and maltreatment, however, clinical aspects of the shortness of breath are also discussed.

Objectives
At the completion of this scenario, the student will be able to:
- Explain the common signs and symptoms attributed to elder abuse.
- Discuss the requirements for reporting suspected elder abuse.
- Describe the signs and symptoms of neglect.

Case Presentation
Your ALS unit is dispatched to the home of a 70-year-old woman who has shortness of breath. You enter the apartment to the smell of garbage and urine. The surroundings are very dirty and remnants of previous meals are scattered on the table. A neighbor, who had not heard from the patient in a long time despite a history of frequent visits in the past, dropped by and found the patient very short of breath. The neighbor called EMS and when you arrive, the patient states that she is "always short of breath" but that she is worse on this occasion. The patient's visitor states that he has not seen the patient in a long time and is not sure of the patient's baseline status.

Faculty Information
Initial Assessment
ABCDEs:
- Airway: The patient's airway is open and there are no signs of obstruction.
- Breathing: The respiratory rate is 24 to 26 breaths/min and the oxygen saturation is 86%. There are bilateral moist crackles on auscultation.
- Circulation: The patient's heart rate is 110 beats/min and irregular, and the blood pressure is 186/118 mm Hg.
- Disability: The patient is alert and is conversant, except for speaking limitations imposed by shortness of breath.
- Exposure: There are no signs of trauma on inspection of the patient.

ALS Information:
- ECG: Atrial fibrillation with uniform premature ventricular contractions at around 4–6/min.
- Blood sugar: 156 mg/dL.
- Temperature: 97.6° F

SAMPLE History:
- Signs: Patient complains of shortness of breath and is speaking in broken sentences. She is sitting in the tripod position.
- Allergies: Sulfa
- Medications: Lasix, K-Dur, Cardizem, Lanoxin
- Past history: CHF, hypertension, atrial fibrillation
- Last meal: Had dinner last night 14 hours ago
- Events leading up: The shortness of breath has been building for several days. She states she had to sleep upright in the chair last night due to the respiratory distress.

Section 3: Scenarios

◆ GEMS diamond:
- G: Patient has had shortness of breath for several days and had to sleep upright last night. History of CHF, hypertension, atrial fibrillation.
- E: Apartment smells of garbage and urine, is dirty, and remnants of previous meal are scattered on table.
- M: Patient takes Lasix, K-Dur, Cardizem, and Lanoxin.
- S: Neighbor reports a decrease in visits with patient. Patient had dinner 14 hours ago.

The patient has evidence of significant shortness of breath and has a history compatible with pulmonary edema.

■ Management Strategies

Based on this patient's presentation, what are the likely causes of the shortness of breath?
- Congestive heart failure is the most likely explanation, based upon both this presentation and the patient's past history. However, other causes of shortness of breath should be considered.
- An acute coronary syndrome can manifest as congestive heart failure (CHF), and thus this patient should be considered as possibly having a coronary event.
- Other causes of shortness of breath (eg, asthma, COPD) can be addressed and probably ruled out based on history and physical exam.

What is the patient's physiologic status?
- The patient has acute respiratory distress, and should be monitored closely for response to oxygen.
- The patient had hypertension and mild tachycardia, which are consistent with congestive heart failure.

What are the initial management and treatment priorities?
- BLS treatment priorities:
  1. As stabilization and transport continue, obtain a more complete history.
  2. Maintain the airway and provide supplemental oxygen.
  3. Monitor blood pressure.
  4. Provide rapid transport and/or assist ALS providers.
  5. Monitor respiratory rate and hemodynamic status and note appearance of any new symptoms.

- ALS treatment priorities:
  1. BLS priorities, plus consider advanced airway maneuvers if the patient's situation deteriorates.
  2. CPAP or BiPAP if available and allowed per local protocol.
  3. Attempt IV access on the way to the receiving hospital.
  4. Consider pharmacologic [nitroglycerin, aspirin, furosemide (Lasix)] management as indicated by the patient condition and as dictated by regional protocols.
  5. Provide ongoing ECG rhythm monitoring, with performance of a 12-lead ECG if available in the specific ALS system.

■ Issues in Management

- The primary issue in this patient's management is the congestive heart failure. Congestive heart failure should be managed with supplemental oxygen, nitroglycerin, aspirin, morphine, and diuretics (as dictated by patient presentation and local protocols), and other supportive care.
- An issue in management which may be just as important as his CHF in the long term relates to the fact that the patient herself did not activate EMS despite being obviously ill. Presumably, if the neighbor had not come by, the patient would still be at home. This suggests the possibility of self-neglect. As in many other instances, the EMS providers are particularly well suited to note relevant history. For example, while patient stabilization is occurring, glance around the patient's living area and see if it is well-kept or cluttered. You can try and determine whether or not the patient is taking care of herself, both for medical and sustenance needs. Given the fact that "a picture is worth a thousand words," you are in particularly good position to evaluate the situation for self-neglect.

Section 3: Scenarios

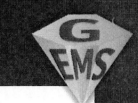

- Assessment for possible self-neglect extends beyond the physical assessment of the patient's living condition. During transport, and assuming the patient's oxygenation status improves such that a history is obtainable, the patient should be asked why she did not activate EMS or see her physician sooner. The patient's responses should be monitored for vague or non-committal reasoning. Be aware of the need to transmit your suspicions of self-neglect to hospital providers who may otherwise be too busy trying to stabilize the patient's CHF to easily recognize the big-picture problem of self neglect.

■ Core Knowledge Points

What is self-neglect?
- Self-neglect is a form of elder abuse. While there may not be actual physical abuse in terms of blunt trauma, neglect can be a serious, if insidious, cause of poor outcome and poor psychological adjustment in older patients.

How can neglect be recognized?
- Neglect patterns can present in similar fashion as other abuse patterns. There can be delays between injury or illness and the seeking of medical attention, or no medical attention initiated by the patient.
- Direct questioning about neglect is not as likely as direct questioning about abuse to yield a concrete determination of neglect. However, questions about the attention patients pay to their own medical care may give indirect and useful information about the potential for neglect.

■ Case Development

This patient had an acute flare of CHF which required hospitalization. The patient did not require intubation, and her oxygen saturation improved easily with supplemental oxygen and medical therapy. The admitting physician involved social services and it was discovered that the patient had had a CHF flare in part because of intermittent adherence with her medical regimen. This was consistent with an overall picture of self-neglect. The patient did not eat right, did not take her medications regularly, and did not express concerns about her symptoms with others, including her physician. Based on the intervention of social services, the patient was provided with a home health assistant, the care of whom markedly reduced further episodes of CHF after hospital discharge.

■ Summary

Patients suffering from elder neglect can be very ill, only coming to medical attention after the intervention of others. They may give vague histories, may only occasionally follow their medication regimen, and may express a low level of interest in the details of taking care of themselves. You are in an excellent position to assess the patient's living environment and report concerns about the potential for neglect to receiving hospital personnel.

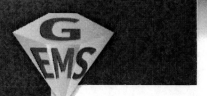

Section 3: Scenarios

ALS Scenarios: Delirium vs. Dementia

This case is designed to facilitate discussion on delirium and dementia. The patient is stable with a recent history of a clinically significant acute change in his mental status. Discussion should be centered on differentiating delirium from dementia.

Objectives

At the completion of this scenario, the student will be able to:
- Discuss the definition of delirium and dementia.
- Distinguish between delirium and dementia.
- Formulate a plan to evaluate the older patient with a complaint related to delirium or dementia.

Case Presentation

It is ten o'clock in the morning and snow is falling. You are working on an ALS ambulance that is dispatched to the home of a man with known Alzheimer's dementia. The patient lives with his daughter and her husband. The daughter states she has noticed a sudden deterioration in the patient's mental status since last night; the patient has decreased attention span and she found him walking in the yard this morning with only his robe on. He is seen monthly by his doctor who had diagnosed the Alzheimer's 6 to 8 months ago. The patient appears disoriented, agitated and also has visual hallucinations. The family reports that these are new symptoms for the patient, whose previous Alzheimer's disease had manifested as a gradual decline in memory and language function over the past half-year.

Faculty Information

Initial Assessment
ABCDEs:
- Airway: The airway is open and there are no signs of obstruction.
- Breathing: Respiratory rate is 18 breaths/min and there are good bilateral breath sounds with an oxygen saturation of 97%.
- Circulation—patient's heart rate is 94 beats/min and the blood pressure is 120/80 mmHg. Skin is warm, pink, and dry.
- Disability: The patient has an apparent alert status but is not oriented. The patient does not respond to questions about person, place and time, but screams at the examiners, asking them why they are trying to hurt him.
- Exposure: There are no signs of trauma on inspection of the patient

SAMPLE History:
- Signs: Due to the patient's disorientation, he is unable to give useful history. The daughter has not noted any signs of acute infection or other problems other than the fact that the patient has had some difficulty sleeping over the past month or two. The primary care physician has told the patient that this problem sleeping is part of the Alzheimer's disease presentation as a possibly depressive manifestation.
- Allergies: No known allergies
- Medications: The daughter states that the primary care physician did not prescribe any specific treatment for the insomnia, but that the patient has been taking sleeping pills (diphenhydramine).
- Past history: Alzheimer's disease
- Last meal: Dinner last night
- Events leading up: Increased disorientation

ALS Information:
- ECG: Normal sinus rhythm without ectopy
- Blood sugar: 110 mg/dL
- Temperature: 97.8° F

Section 3: Scenarios

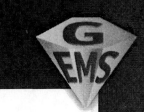

▼ GEMS diamond:
- G: Patient has Alzheimer's dementia, experienced sudden deterioration in mental status.
- E: Nothing noted.
- M: Patient is taking sleeping pills (diphenhydramine).
- S: Patient lives with his daughter and her husband. Daughter noticed deterioration.

The patient has no evidence of physical trauma and there is little available history to suggest metabolic or septic explanations for the symptoms. However, the patient's deterioration seems to be more acute and not characteristic of his baseline Alzheimer's status.

▪ Management Strategies

Based on this patient's presentation, what are the likely causes for the acute deterioration in mental status?
- The patient could have a toxic (drug related), metabolic (electrolyte imbalance), or neurologic (CNS infection or trauma) cause for the apparent delirium. Other causes are also possible; in fact, there are so many causes of acute delirium that further history will be required to narrow down the possibilities.

What is the patient's status?
- The patient is hemodynamically stable and does not appear to have any acute life threats, but serious metabolic, toxic, or CNS abnormalities cannot be ruled out.

What are your initial management and treatment priorities?
- The patient is so agitated and delirious that any advanced life support interventions (such as starting an IV) are essentially impossible. Therefore, the basic treatment priority for both BLS and ALS providers is supportive therapy for the delirium; this will consist of providing a calm, stable environment.

- **If ALS treatment is a possibility, the treatment priorities are:**
  1. Intravenous access
  2. Fluid resuscitation for any signs of dehydration
  3. Pharmacologic interventions either for dementia (see below) or for other conditions (such as hypoglycemia)
  4. Ongoing monitoring of vital signs and ECG rhythm

▪ Issues in Management

- The primary issue in management is calming the patient to the point that further therapies can be instituted. Regardless of the cause of altered mental status, a priority should be getting the patient to a point where further ALS interventions are possible.
- Balance the desire to provide stabilization with the fact that aggressive moves towards the patient could result in exacerbation of the delirious state, and even injury to the patient.
- Besides general supportive measures, specific issues in management may relate to various causes of delirium. Electrolyte replacement, glucose replacement, correction of arrhythmias, or treatment of congestive heart failure may help patients with delirium.

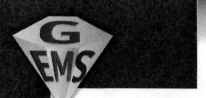

Section 3: Scenarios

■ Core Knowledge Points

What is supportive therapy for delirium?
- Non-pharmacologic management includes treating any specific causes as well as trying to keep the patient quiet and minimizing excessive stimulation.
- Having family members or familiar faces is helpful in the prehospital setting, and you should encourage these individuals to accompany the patient to the hospital.
- Communicate in a simple and direct, yet nonthreatening, style.
- Physical restraints should only be used as a last resort, as this can endanger patient cooperation, be counterproductive for patient safety, and cause injury to the older patient's fragile skin. However, in some cases, patient safety will be maintained by use of restraints. Check your local protocol regarding the use of restraints.

What is the pharmacologic management of delirium?
- Depending on capabilities and protocols, the following medications may be used:
  1. Haloperidol
  2. Lorazepam or other benzodiazepine
- Specific pharmacologic management occurs only after supportive therapy (see above) has been utilized.

How is your interaction with the patient critical in delirium management?
- Your response to the emergency is the patient's first interaction with the medical system in its evaluation of his or her delirium. EMS providers can make a good first impression on the patient, setting them up for a positive experience. Employ a direct and gentle approach with minimal stimulation and maximal understanding of the patient's condition and confused state. Your correct approach both calms the patient and minimizes fears of the visit to the receiving hospital.

■ Case Development

Based on the history of the patient's difficulty sleeping, and information from the family members regarding the patient's medications, a diphenhydramine-containing sleep aid was found. While the patient was not able to give a detailed history, he was able to confirm that he had been taking a number of the sleeping pills. The paramedics brought this medication with them to the receiving institution, where the work up ultimately yielded a diagnosis of diphenhydramine-associated delirium.

■ Summary

Like dementia, delirium has a number of causes, but delirium must also be differentiated from the more long-standing condition of dementia. Since disorientation is a hallmark of delirium, emphasize a calm and understanding approach in initial evaluation of these patients. Such supportive therapy improves the chances of getting an improved history and providing a definitive therapy, if one exists.

Complicating the fact that delirium is sometimes difficult to differentiate from dementia is the fact that, as in this case, delirium can occur in a patient with known dementia. In fact, Alzheimer's dementia is a well-known risk factor for development of a secondary delirious state.

Skill Stations

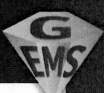

Section 4

David L. Seabrook, MPA, EMT-P
Antonio Suarez, MSA, NREMT-P

Contents

- **Skill Station Overview** **186**
- **BLS and ALS Skill Stations** **188**
    - Conducting a Patient Assessment Interview 188
    - Immobilization 209
- **Optional ALS Skill Station** **224**
    - Intravenous Therapy 224

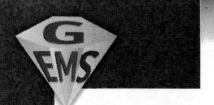

Section 4: Skill Stations

Skill Station Overview

There are two required Skill Stations in the GEMS course. Station 1 is on conducting a patient assessment interview, and Station 2 covers immobilization of an older patient. The stations apply to both a BLS and an ALS audience.

This section also contains an optional ALS skill station on Intravenous Therapy. This skill can be presented if you wish to run a longer, more comprehensive ALS course.

To successfully prepare for and run the stations, ensure that you do the following.

Before the course:
- Ensure that you have enough room to conduct the skill stations. You will need breakout rooms capable of holding 6 students and 1 instructor, plus the equipment for each station to be run.
- Ensure that you have collected the equipment prior to the course. See the list of equipment for each skill in the following two sections. If you are using the Catalyst® Geriatric Simulation Kit, make sure you have enough kits to go around. If you will be making the required equipment, note that some of it will need attention before the start of the course. Note that this includes making photocopies of the observer handouts for each simulation. Role-play instructions are provided in the GEMS Teaching Package for convenience.
- Read the following pages regarding how the skill stations should run. These pages also provide key information and teaching points that will prepare you for discussion.

During the course:
- At the beginning of the day during registration, assign a group number to each individual. This number will be used later to efficiently organize the students into their skill station and scenario groups.
- When it is time to begin the first skill session, divide the students into smaller groups for instruction according to the group numbers assigned to them during registration. Assign each group to one of the smaller breakout rooms.
- Once in the small groups, the Faculty introduce the station and give a brief overview of what should be done during the skill station.
- Assign a role to each student in the station and hand out the role-play instructions to the students assigned those roles. Be sure to hand out the "Observer" sheet to the assigned observers. The role of the observers is critical in the post-simulation discussion. Have them discuss their responses to the questions; oftentimes they provide valuable insight to the students who played the roles.
- Be sure to ask the student playing the patient how he or she felt during the simulation. The students playing the providers may think that they communicated appropriately with the patient, when in fact they did not. This is a teachable moment in which students can learn a great deal from pointers on how to better communicate.
- Supervise the students during the simulations. Provide information such as vital signs when requested. If a student asks a question that is not answered in these Faculty materials, provide an answer that you feel to be appropriate based on the case.
- Actively manage the amount of time spent on each skill so that there is enough time for 2 to 3 simulations within the allotted timeframe. Do not let students become sidetracked by irrelevant issues.

Notes on Skill Station 1: Conducting a Patient Assessment Interview
- During Station 1, conduct 2 to 3 simulations to allow as many students as possible to play the patient. An option after completing Situation 1 is to allow all students to try on the simulation materials such as the glasses, hearing aids, and mouth guards or the materials in the Catalyst® Geriatric Simulation Kit at the end of the skill station or as part of your discussion of the patient's needs and how they were handled.
- Consider having the students wear the simulation glasses and hearing aids during part of their lunch break. This will give them another chance to experience first-hand the difficulties that older people face on a daily basis.

Section 4: Skill Stations

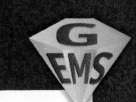

■ Notes on Skill Station 2: Immobilization

- Simulating kyphosis on a young person can be difficult, but is important in this skill. A towel or football can be placed below the student's neck inside their shirt. Advise the student playing the patient to keep his or her head and shoulders flexed forward during the skill if possible. Bring an old T-shirt to the skill station so that the student's own shirt does not get stretched out. If a geriatric manikin is available, consider using it for this skill to demonstrate head immobilization of a kyphotic patient.
- The video component of the course shows how to immobilize a kyphotic patient. You may also consider demonstrating this skill at the beginning of the skill station to emphasize the major points if time allows.
- Students simulating the patient should wear the patient simulation materials, such as the glasses and earplugs, in this skill as well, so they can experience what it is like to be older, and so the students playing the EMS providers can practice communication skills.

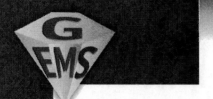

Section 4: Skill Stations

Skill Station #1: Conducting a Patient Assessment Interview

This 45-minute skill station will allow BLS and ALS students to practice "hands-on" assessment and interview skills. Three emergency situations are provided for use in this skill station.

Objectives

At the end of this station, the student will be able to:
- Direct each scenario in a systematic, consistent way using standard EMS assessment skills.
- Recognize the importance of proper communication techniques.
- Recognize the importance of history-taking in the older patient.
- Organize a comprehensive exam to determine the basis for the patient's symptoms.
- Show a balanced approach to integrate the physical exam with history-taking.

Format

Student-Faculty ratio: six students per one Faculty member.

For each of the communication and assessment scenarios, one student will serve as the coached patient-actor. One will act as a coached family member-actor or police officer-actor if applicable. Two students will serve as the responding EMS crew. The remaining students will be observers and assist with the post-assessment critique led by the Faculty.

Logistics

Station: 45 minutes
Breakdown:

3 min.	Faculty introduces format and expectations.
2 min.	**Situation #1:**
	1st patient-actor taken aside, coached. Family member coached.
8 min.	Rescue crew assesses/interviews patient.
3 min.	Debriefing, critique
2 min.	**Situation #2:**
	2nd patient-actor chosen, taken aside, coached. Police officer coached.
8 min.	2nd rescue crew assesses/interviews patient.
3 min.	Debriefing, critique
2 min.	**Situation #3:**
	3rd patient-actor chosen, taken aside, coached.
8 min.	3rd rescue crew assesses/interviews patient.
3 min.	Debriefing, critique
3 min.	Wrap-up

Room Requirements

The room should be large enough to hold six students, the Faculty, and all the carry-in EMS equipment. The room should be quiet enough to permit interviewing and listening. There should be a chair for the simulated patient placed centrally, and enough other chairs and tables to accommodate the other students. There should be enough room around the patient for two rescuers to work.

Equipment Needs

Notecards for simulation (provided in GEMS Teaching Package and in this section)
Exam gloves (1 box each of large, medium, and small) (latex-free if possible)
Oxygen tank and oxygen administration supplies

Section 4: Skill Stations

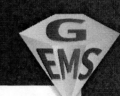

First aid kit including blood pressure cuff, stethoscope
Medication bottles with simulated labels (hydrochlorthiazide, nitroglycerin, furosemide, and potassium)
Ziploc bags
Mouth guards or large gumballs (Note: For the course, you will need one mouth guard or gumball per student. If you opt to use the Additional Activities found on page 190, you will need additional mouth guards/gumballs.)
Earplugs (Note: For the course, you will need one pair of earplugs per student in total. If you opt to use the Additional Activities found on page 190, you will need additional pairs of earplugs.)
Patient simulation materials:
- Sunglasses with tape on lenses (can be plastic, nonprescription)
- Yellow-tinted (or other color) sunglasses

Or

- Geriatric simulation kit

Tattered clothes/robes
Winter coat

Equipment for Additional Activities

The Additional Activities are discussed on page 190. If you opt to use the Additional Activities, you will need to obtain the following additional supplies.
- Earplugs
- Mouth guards or large gumballs
- Stones/pebbles (to put in shoes)
- Gauze and tape (to tape hands to practice impaired mobility)
- RMA forms (to practice signing with impaired mobility)
- Small pill-sized candies (such as Tic-Tacs) in assorted colors, placed in a medication bottle
- Photocopies of page from business section of phone book.
- Dishwashing gloves to simulate arthritis or coordination problems (only required if you are not using the Catalyst® Geriatric Simulation Kit)

Teaching Points

The Faculty will cover the following points during this skill station. Standard EMS assessment technique should be followed; however, the following should be considered in assessing the older patient:
- Communication should be tailored to the patient's needs.
- History-taking requires greater skill when dealing with a patient who has communication difficulties.
- In-depth questioning may be needed to gain an understanding of the patient's past medical history.
- Questioning of family and caregivers may help uncover important information.
- Patient's medications should be carefully documented and/or transported with the patient.
- Thorough physical examination may help reveal problems other than the chief complaint.

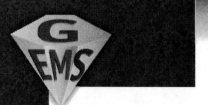

Section 4: Skill Stations

Additional Activities

An option during Skill Station 1 is to, after completing Situation 1, have all students try on the glasses, mouth guards, and ear plugs, or the materials in the Catalyst® Geriatric Simulation Kit. In order to complete the experience, the Faculty should act as a responding EMS provider and offer each student one obstacle to overcome.

For this option, collect the following additional equipment beforehand:
- Small pill-sized candies (such as Tic-Tacs) in assorted colors, placed in a medication bottle
- Standard local phone book (must include residential/business listing, not just yellow pages)
- Dishwashing gloves to simulate arthritis or coordination problems (if not using the Catalyst® Geriatric Simulation Kit)

The following activities may be performed by the students during this segment of the skill station:
1. Ask a student to open a medicine bottle while wearing gloves to simulate arthritis.
2. Ask a student to select a certain color pill while wearing glasses to simulate vision problems. ***Note to instructor: In this instance, fill the medicine bottle with Tic-Tacs or other small (pill-sized) candy of different colors prior to the course.***
3. Ask a student to tell you his or her medical history. While the student is doing this, avoid making eye contact, and look around the room instead. Also, when you speak to the student, avoid talking in his or her direction.
4. Give one student a mouth guard and a list of medications. Ask the student what medications he or she is on, and repeat back exactly what you hear (pretend you do not know about these medications and are trying to obtain a list).
5. Ask a student to look up the name of a doctor (so you can talk to the doctor) in the business section of a phone book (to address reading smaller type with vision problems).
6. Have a student sign an RMA form while wearing gloves and glasses, to simulate arthritis and vision problems.

When the students have each had a turn completing a task, allow them to share what they felt with the group. Do they think that there is a better way to get a history? Are there better ways to communicate?

After completing this part of the skill, move on to Scenario 2 and complete it if time permits.

Section 4: Skill Stations

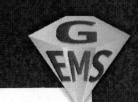

Situation #1

In Situation #1, one student simulates the patient, one student simulates a family member, two students simulate the EMS team, and the remaining students serve as observers.

On the following page, directions for each of the simulated parties are provided. These directions are provided as perforated cards in the GEMS Teaching Package for convenience. If you do not have the GEMS Teaching Package, before you teach the course, photocopy the instructions for each situation and cut them at the dotted lines. Distribute these to the students. Be sure to make enough photocopies for two skill sessions.

Give the glasses, earplugs, and wheelchair (if available) to the student simulating the patient.

Hand the dispatch information to one of the observing students to read out loud when you are ready to begin.

Tell the students to begin. Announce that they have 8 minutes to complete the call.

Half way through the call, announce that they are half way. Make a subsequent announcement when there are 2 minutes left.

Section 4: Skill Stations

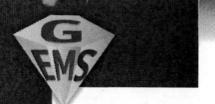

CONDUCTING A PATIENT ASSESSMENT INTERVIEW
Situation 1

Simulated Patient:

You will be a 78-year-old woman (or man) who lives at home alone. You are normally alert and able to care for yourself. Your son (or daughter) while visiting you this morning noticed that you are weak, and you seem out of breath. You should answer questions appropriately, but with a few seconds delay between the question and your answer. You should simulate a slightly elevated respiratory rate. Your chief complaint is vague, you feel weak, "just can't seem to get going," "legs feel shaky," etc. You deny chest pain. <u>IF</u> specifically asked, you admit to slight shortness of breath. <u>IF</u> asked about medical history, you give a vague answer of an unknown heart problem. You deny recent illness/injury.

Props: The Faculty will provide you with glasses to simulate vision problems and earplugs to simulate hearing problems. If available, a wheelchair will be provided for you to sit in.

CONDUCTING A PATIENT ASSESSMENT INTERVIEW
Situation 1

Simulated Family Member:

Your Mom (or Dad) is normally quite alert. She/he ambulates with a cane. She/he has a history of hypertension and angina. She/he takes medicines for this (hydrochlorthiazide and nitro) as well as a "water pill" (furosemide) and potassium. She/he has an allergy to penicillin.

When EMS arrives, you answer the door and lead them to your parent.

CONDUCTING A PATIENT ASSESSMENT INTERVIEW
Situation 1

EMS Team:

You will be asked to assess and treat a simulated patient. As much as possible, obtain your information from the patient. Use a hands-on approach to this training exercise. Certain assessment information will be provided to you as your assessment progresses. For example, if you apply a BP cuff and simulate its inflation, you will be provided with the simulated blood pressure. At the conclusion of your assessment, you will be asked to provide a brief "radio style" report on your patient.

CONDUCTING A PATIENT ASSESSMENT INTERVIEW
Situation 1

Dispatch Information:

You are a BLS (ALS) ambulance responding to a 78-year-old woman (man) for weakness at 12:30 pm. You arrive to a modest but clean home in an older neighborhood. The scene appears safe and you are greeted at the door by a younger person who takes you to the patient.

Section 4: Skill Stations

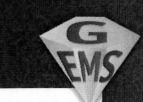

CONDUCTING A PATIENT ASSESSMENT INTERVIEW
Situation 1

Observing Students:
Your role in this situation is to observe the providers responding to the simulated call. Throughout the call, pay particular attention to what the providers did or did not do to address the patient's communication issues. As you are observing the call, fill out the following questions:

1. Did the providers try to speak with the patient?   _____ Yes   _____ No

_____

_____

2. How many attempts did they make to communicate with the patient before turning their focus to the family member?

_____

_____

3. Did they wait longer than usual for the patient to answer?

_____

_____

4. Were they creative in finding ways to get the patient to communicate? If not, what else could they have done?

_____

_____

5. How did the patient react to the way the providers were interacting with him or her? Do you think that the patient understood what the providers were saying and doing? From the patient's standpoint, were his or her emotional needs met?

_____

_____

When the situation is finished, report your observances to the group.

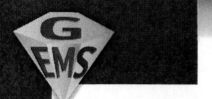

Section 4: Skill Stations

Initial Assessment/Focused History and Physical Exam

In this chart, information regarding the patient is provided in regular font. This information should be given to the students simulating the EMS crew if they ask for it. Possible interventions are provided in italics.

Assessment	Actions, Findings, and *Possible Interventions*
Scene Safety • The scene appears safe. • Providers take BSI precautions.	
Initial Assessment • Providers introduce selves.	*Providers determine relation of younger person to patient. Providers properly position themselves at patient's level for direct communication. Providers address vision and communication problems by speaking at a slower pace and showing a caring manner.* Initial impression of patient: conscious, pale, lethargic
• Airway	Airway is open.
• Breathing	Breathing is rapid—approximately 28 breaths/min. *Administer supplemental oxygen. With supplemental oxygen, the patient's mentation seems a little clearer. (Check pulse oximetry level if possible.)*
• Circulation	Pulse is strong, slightly elevated.
• Mental status	Patient answers questions appropriately but slowly. *Providers should ask about normal mentation, speech patterns.*

Focused History & Physical Exam
• Providers check vital signs:
  • Blood pressure
  • Pulse
  • Respirations
  • Lung sounds
  • Temperature
  • Pulse oximetry (if not already checked)
  • Glucose level
	
	BP = 114/62 mm Hg
	HR = 110 beats/min
	RR = 28 breaths/min
	Lung sounds = abnormal (fine basilar crackles)
	Temp = 97.2°F
	SpO_2 = 92% on room air/ 96% on O_2
	BG = 92 mg/dL

• Providers ask pertinent questions of patient <u>and</u> patient's son (daughter).	Information obtained should include the SAMPLE history: • Signs and Symptoms: Weakness, short of breath • Allergies: Penicillin • Medications: Hydrochlorthiazide (HCTZ), nitro-tabs, furosemide, potassium supplements • Past medical history: Hypertension and angina • Last intake: Lunch $1/2$ hour ago • Events leading up: Shortness of breath occasionally, but the weakness is new this morning

Section 4: Skill Stations

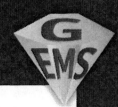

- Providers apply cardiac monitor.

  Cardiac monitor shows sinus tachycardia, QRS complexes are slightly widened.

- Providers perform 12-lead ECG.

  ECG shows ST elevation in lateral leads.

Management Strategies

What are your initial treatment priorities?

BLS priorities:
- Provide O$_2$.
- Carefully interview patient and caregiver to search for the cause of weakness.
- Maintain high index of suspicion for MI and/or a septic problem.

ALS priorities:
- BLS priorities plus:
  - Start an IV.
  - Monitor ECG.
  - Maintain high index of suspicion for MI and/or a septic problem.
  - Check 12-lead ECG if available.

If MI diagnosed by ALS crew:
- Administer aspirin.
- Depending on local protocol, treatment with nitroglycerin and/or furosemide may be indicated.
- Consider prioritized transport to a cardiac care hospital.

GEMS diamond:
- G: Patient feels weak, shaky, and has no chest pain. Unknown heart problem.
- E: Home is modest but clean. Patient ambulates with a cane.
- M: Patient takes hydrochlorthiazide, nitro, water pill, and potassium.
- S: Patient lives at home alone. Son (daughter) visits.

Issues in Management

This case first of all represents a communication challenge. Communication with older patient may require patience and will be facilitated by good technique. Direct positioning of the provider in front of the patient and using a clear and adequate voice level will help. Also, the EMS team should designate a single provider to ask questions of the patient rather than having questions come from multiple directions.

This case also shows an atypical presentation of myocardial infarction. In persons older than age 75 who are having an MI, the presentation is more likely to be shortness of breath rather than classic chest pain. EMS providers should maintain a high index of suspicion for MI in the older patient who presents with acute functional decline, dyspnea, syncope, falls, or acute confusion.

Case Development

As mentioned earlier, with supplemental oxygen, the patient's mentation seems a little clearer. Transport occurs without event.

Core Knowledge Points

At the end of the call, tell the EMS team to provide a brief "radio style" report on the patient. After this is complete, ask the two observers to each give a report on what they observed during the call, and to specifically address the questions that they were asked to fill out on their form.

Section 4: Skill Stations

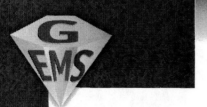

Pay particular attention to the patient's account of how the call went versus the provider's accounts of the call. Is there disparity between the two accounts? Many times, even when the providers truly believe that they communicated effectively with the patient, the patient feels differently. Point this out in class. Give pointers for how the providers could have communicated effectively with the older patient. Solicit advice from the student who played the patient; he or she may have valuable suggestions regarding what did and did not work, as well as suggestions for what could have been done differently. This is a teachable moment—this is where students can really learn how they come across and what they can do differently. This discussion should provide them with memorable, real, practical advice that they can use in the field.

What is good technique for interviewing an older patient?
- Direct questioning of the patient is the primary choice.
- Correlating and background information may be obtained from family or caregivers.
- Correct positioning in the patient's line of sight and adequate voice tone are important.
- Allow adequate time for answers to questions.
- Avoid multiple questioners.

What are the ways that MI can present atypically in the older patient?
- Shortness of breath
- Non-classic pain, discomfort, numbness
- Acute onset weakness, confusion, or functional decline

What is the best way to discover an atypically presenting MI?
- Careful, deliberate, thorough history-taking
- Thorough physical exam including electrocardiography

Summary

This case illustrates the assessment of an older patient with the vague but common complaint of weakness. While weakness could have many causes, one of the most significant if missed is myocardial ischemia/infarction. A provider who performs a thorough exam and takes a careful history will help patients survive these events with the least possible damage.

Section 4: Skill Stations

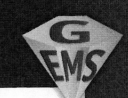

Situation #2

In Situation #2, one student simulates the patient, one student simulates the police, two students simulate the EMS team, and the remaining students serve as observers.

On the following page, directions for each of the simulated parties are provided. These directions are provided as perforated cards in the GEMS Teaching Package for convenience. If you do not have the GEMS Teaching Package, before you teach the course, photocopy the instructions for each situation and cut them at the dotted lines. Distribute these to the students. Be sure to make enough photocopies for two skill sessions.

Give the glasses, a mouth guard or gumball, and tattered clothes to the student simulating the patient.

Hand the dispatch information to one of the observing students to read out loud when you are ready to begin.

Tell the students to begin. Announce that they have 8 minutes to complete the call.

Half way through the call, announce that they are half way. Make a subsequent announcement when there are 2 minutes left.

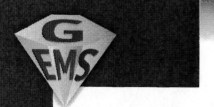

Section 4: Skill Stations

CONDUCTING A PATIENT ASSESSMENT INTERVIEW
Situation 2

Simulated Patient:
You will be a 63-year-old man (or woman) who lives at home with a spouse. You are normally alert and able to care for yourself. You have dementia secondary to Alzheimer's disease and answer questions inappropriately. You should simulate a disoriented patient. Your chief complaint is "I can't remember who I am" and you deny chest pain or a headache. Your spouse is out shopping for groceries. <u>IF</u> asked about medical history, you give a vague answer, denying recent illness or injury. <u>IF</u> asked, you remember that you did not take your medication this morning.

Props: The Faculty will provide you with tattered clothes. Prepare yourself as an ungroomed patient. Hair should be messy and clothing improperly applied (inside out, buttons misaligned). The instructor will also provide you with glasses to simulate vision problems and a mouth guard or gumball to simulate speech impairment.

CONDUCTING A PATIENT ASSESSMENT INTERVIEW
Situation 2

EMS Team:
You will be asked to assess and treat a simulated patient. As much as possible, obtain your information from the patient. Use a hands-on approach to this training exercise. Certain assessment information will be provided to you as your assessment progresses. For example, if you apply a BP cuff and simulate its inflation, you will be provided with the simulated blood pressure. At the conclusion of your assessment, you will be asked to provide a brief "radio style" report on your patient.

CONDUCTING A PATIENT ASSESSMENT INTERVIEW
Situation 2

Police Officer:
You were called to the scene by the patient because the patient could not remember who he or she was. You were trying to locate the patient's spouse, and then called EMS when you noticed that the patient was talking to himself/herself and occasionally answering questions inappropriately. You have been keeping the patient company while waiting for the EMS team. <u>IF</u> the EMS team asks you about your interaction with the patient, tell them that the patient said he or she is afraid of going to the hospital because the house could be robbed. <u>IF</u> the EMS team asks you to help with any aspect of the call, do so.

When EMS arrives, you answer the door and lead them to the patient.

CONDUCTING A PATIENT ASSESSMENT INTERVIEW
Situation 2

Dispatch Information:
You are a BLS (ALS) ambulance dispatched to the private residence of a 63-year-old man (woman). Police are there because the patient called the precinct and stated "I can't recall who I am." Police were investigating the whereabouts of the spouse and during their conversation noticed that the patient was talking to himself/herself and occasionally answered questions inappropriately. The police called EMS to respond.

When you arrive, a police officer answers the door and leads you to the patient, who is half dressed and looking disheveled. The scene appears safe.

Section 4: Skill Stations

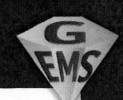

CONDUCTING A PATIENT ASSESSMENT INTERVIEW
Situation 2

Observing Students:
Your role in this situation is to observe the providers responding to the simulated call. Throughout the call, pay particular attention to what the providers did or did not do to address the patient's communication issues. As you are observing the call, fill out the following questions:

1. Did the providers try to speak with the patient? _____ Yes _____ No

_____

_____

2. How many attempts did they make to communicate with the patient before giving up, or turning their attention elsewhere?

_____

_____

3. Did they wait longer than usual for the patient to answer?

_____

_____

4. Were they creative in finding ways to get the patient to communicate? If not, what else could they have done?

_____

_____

5. How did the patient react to the way the providers were interacting with him or her? Do you think that the patient understood what the providers were saying and doing? From the patient's standpoint, were his or her emotional needs met?

_____

_____

When the situation is finished, report your observances to the group.

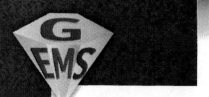

Section 4: Skill Stations

Initial Assessment/Focused History and Physical Exam

In this chart, information regarding the patient is provided in regular font. This information should be given to the students simulating the EMS crew if they ask for it. Possible interventions are provided in italics.

Assessment	Actions, Findings, and *Possible Interventions*
Scene Safety • The scene appears safe. • Providers take BSI precautions. • The environment feels hot.	*Have the police stay, in case the patient becomes violent or a potentially unsafe situation develops.*
Initial Assessment • Providers introduce selves.	*Providers properly position themselves at patient's level for direct communication. Providers address vision and communication problems by speaking at a slower pace and showing a caring manner.* Initial impression of patient: conscious, disoriented.
• Airway	Airway is open.
• Breathing	Breathing is normal—approximately 18 breaths/min. *Administer supplemental oxygen. (Check pulse oximetry level if possible.)*
• Circulation	Pulse is strong, within normal limits.
• Mental status	Patient answers questions inappropriately and seems to be forgetful. *Providers should ask about normal mentation, speech patterns. Assessment of cognitive function such as orientation to person, place, and time; perception of reality, presence of disorganized thought, evidence of delusions, hallucinations and disorganized speech are all significant findings.*

Focused History & Physical Exam
• Providers check vital signs:
  • Blood pressure
  • Pulse
  • Respirations
  • Lung sounds
  • Temperature
  • Pulse oximetry (if not already checked)
  • Glucose level
	BP = 114/62 mm Hg
	HR = 88 beats/min
	RR = 18 breaths/min
	Lung sounds = clear bilaterally
	Temp = 98.6°F
	SpO_2 = 98% on room air/ 100% on O_2
	BG = 92 mg/dL

• Providers ask pertinent questions of patient.	Information obtained should include the SAMPLE history: • Signs and Symptoms: Patient makes no complaints other than that he cannot remember who he is. • Allergies: Unknown • Medications: Aricept is found in the bathroom cabinet after searching. • Past medical history: Patient is wearing medical bracelet that indicates a history of Alzheimer's disease. • Last intake: Unknown. • Events leading up: Unknown.

Section 4: Skill Stations

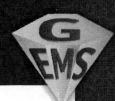

• Providers apply cardiac monitor.	Cardiac monitor and 12-lead ECG show 1st degree heart block.
• Providers perform 12-lead ECG.	

Management Strategies

What are your initial treatment priorities?

BLS priorities:
- Provide O_2.
- Carefully interview patient to search for the cause of disorientation (AMS).
- Maintain a high index of suspicion for medication non-adherence or abuse.
- If hypoglycemia is suspected and the patient is conscious, oral glucose can be administered.

ALS priorities:
- BLS priorities plus:
  - Start an IV.
  - Maintain a high index of suspicion for altered mental status due to hypoglycemia, hyperglycemia, and hypoxia, which are temporary and curable.

If hypoglycemia is diagnosed by ALS crew:
- Administer dextrose, thiamine (depending on local medical direction).
- Consider transport to an emergency department.

If narcotic use is diagnosed by ALS crew:
- Administer naloxone (depending on local medical direction).
- Consider transport to an emergency department.
- ◆ GEMS diamond:
  - G: Patient has dementia, Alzheimer's disease, no chest pain, no headache, and is disoriented.
  - E: Nothing noted.
  - M: Patient did not take medication this morning. Aricept is found in medicine cabinet.
  - S: Patient lives at home with spouse. Spouse is not present.

Issues in Management

A behavioral emergency may represent a threat to the well-being of an older patient. Such behavior may also represent a threat to the well-being or life of another. In this case, scene safety is imperative; if the scene becomes violent, you should have police present during your evaluation. Look for signs of general environmental conditions, and any clue that indicates a previously existing medical problem, such as diabetes.

Also, it is important to remember to protect the patient's privacy. When arriving at the scene, consider turning off your ambulance lights and lowering your radio if allowed by protocol. Calling EMS for help can be embarrassing for older people. Minimizing the amount of attention you draw can help the call to run more smoothly.

Case Development

The patient remembers that he (she) didn't take his (her) medication this morning.

Core Knowledge Points

At the end of the call, tell the EMS team to provide a brief "radio style" report on the patient. After this is complete, ask the two observers to each give a report on what they observed during the call, and to specifically address the questions that they were asked to fill out on their form.

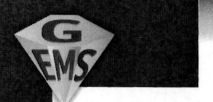

Section 4: Skill Stations

Pay particular attention to the patient's account of how the call went versus the providers accounts of the call. Is there disparity between the two accounts? Many times, even when the providers truly believe that they communicated effectively with the patient, the patient feels differently. Point this out in class. Give pointers for how the providers could have communicated effectively with the older patient. Solicit advice from the student who played the patient; he or she may have valuable suggestions regarding what did and did not work, as well as suggestions for what could have been done differently. This is a teachable moment—this is where students can really learn how they come across and what they can do differently. This discussion should provide them with memorable, real, practical advice that they can use in the field.

What is good technique for interviewing an older patient?
- Direct questioning of the patient is the primary choice.
- Correlating and background information may be obtained from family or caregivers.
- Correct positioning in the patient's line of sight and adequate voice tone are important.
- Allow adequate time for answers to questions.
- Avoid multiple questioners.

Summary

This case illustrates the assessment of an older patient with dementia due to Alzheimer's disease, which has an organic cause and specifically is known to affect the older population. This degenerative and progressive disease causes profound impairment in cognitive abilities, whereas delirium is grossly impaired cognition caused by "organic brain syndrome" associated with fever, hypermetabolic states, and drug withdrawals. Delirium is a condition with a specific cause that can be treated and reversed, unlike dementia, which is degenerative and progressively gets worse with time. A provider who performs a thorough exam and takes a careful history will help patients with these events, preventing any harm to the patient and the providers .The provider's role in these cases is usually supportive.

Section 4: Skill Stations

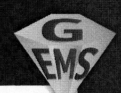

Situation #3

In Situation #3, one student simulates the patient, two students simulate the EMS team, and three students serve as observers.

On the following page, directions for each of the simulated parties are provided. These directions are provided as perforated cards in the GEMS Teaching Package for convenience. If you do not have the GEMS Teaching Package, before you teach the course, photocopy the instructions for each situation and cut them at the dotted lines. Distribute these to the students. Be sure to make enough photocopies for two skill sessions.

Give the glasses, earplugs, a heavy winter coat, and multiple layers of clothes to the student simulating the patient.

Hand the dispatch information to one of the observing students to read out loud when you are ready to begin.

Tell the students to begin. Announce that they have 8 minutes to complete the call.

Half way through the call, announce that they are half way. Make a subsequent announcement when there are 2 minutes left.

Section 4: Skill Stations

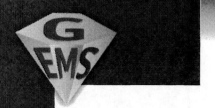

CONDUCTING A PATIENT ASSESSMENT INTERVIEW
Situation 3

Simulated Patient:

You will be an 84-year-old woman (or man) who lives at home alone. You are alert and oriented. You have a persistent productive cough and state to the providers, "This cold hasn't gone away in two weeks." This scenario occurs in the winter—the outdoor temperature is 20°F. The temperature inside the residence is a frigid 38°F. _IF_ asked, you also state that you are depressed over the death of your spouse and don't care about anything.

When EMS arrives, you cough and tell them to come in.

Props: The Faculty will provide you with a heavy winter coat and multiple layers of clothes. Put these on to prepare yourself as a patient wearing multiple layers of clothes to stay warm. The instructor will also provide you with glasses to simulate vision problems and ear plugs to simulate hearing problems.

CONDUCTING A PATIENT ASSESSMENT INTERVIEW
Situation 3

EMS Team:

You will be asked to assess and treat a simulated patient. As much as possible, obtain your information from the patient. Use a hands-on approach to this training exercise. Certain assessment information will be provided to you as your assessment progresses. For example, if you apply a BP cuff and simulate its inflation, you will be provided with the simulated blood pressure. At the conclusion of your assessment, you will be asked to provide a brief "radio style" report on your patient.

Upon arrival, you hear audible coughing coming from inside the residence. You notice newspapers and mail stacked up against the door outside. The scene appears safe.

CONDUCTING A PATIENT ASSESSMENT INTERVIEW
Situation 3

Dispatch Information:

You are a BLS (ALS) ambulance dispatched to the private residence of an 84-year-old woman (man) with persistent coughing—unknown medical.

Section 4: Skill Stations

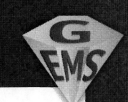

CONDUCTING A PATIENT ASSESSMENT INTERVIEW
Situation 3

Observing Students:
Your role in this situation is to observe the providers responding to the simulated call. Throughout the call, pay particular attention to what the providers did or did not do to address the patient's living circumstances. As you are observing the call, fill out the following questions:

1. Did the providers try to speak with the patient?   _____ Yes   _____ No

_____

_____

2. How many attempts did they make to communicate with the patient before giving up, or turning their attention elsewhere?

_____

_____

3. Did they ask questions about the patient's living conditions, such as why the heat is off?

_____

_____

4. Were they creative in finding ways to get the patient to communicate? If not, what else could they have done? Did they get the patient to talk about his/her depression?

_____

_____

5. How did the patient react to the way the providers were interacting with him or her? Do you think that the patient understood what the providers were saying and doing? From the patient's standpoint, were his or her emotional needs met?

_____

_____

When the situation is finished, report your observances to the group.

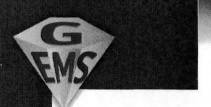

Section 4: Skill Stations

Initial Assessment/Focused History and Physical Exam

In this chart, information regarding the patient is provided in regular font. This information should be given to the students simulating the EMS crew if they ask for it. Possible interventions are provided in italics.

Assessment	Actions, Findings, and *Possible Interventions*
Scene Safety • The scene appears safe. • Providers take BSI precautions.	Inside the home, it is 38°F. The patient's breath is visible due to the cold temperature of the room. It appears that the heat is off. The residence is filthy.
Initial Assessment • Providers introduce selves.	*Providers properly position themselves at patient's level for direct communication. Providers address vision and communication problems by speaking at a slower pace and showing a caring manner.* Initial impression of patient: Alert, oriented, and depressed.
• Airway	Airway is open.
• Breathing	Breathing is tachypnic—approximately 30 breaths/min. Lung sounds are abnormal (rhonchi). *Administer supplemental oxygen.* There is no shortness of breath. *(Check pulse oximetry level if possible.)*
• Circulation	Pulse is strong, within normal limits.
• Mental status	Patient answers questions appropriately and coughs intermittently during your assessment and interview. *Providers should ask about how long patient has had a productive cough. Assessment of cognitive function such as orientation to person, place, and time should be conducted.*
Focused History & Physical Exam • Providers check vital signs:	
• Blood pressure	BP = 140/80 mm Hg
• Pulse	HR = 80 beats/min
• Respirations	RR = 30 breaths/min
• Lung sounds	Lung sounds = abnormal (diffused rhonchi)
• Temperature	Temp = 102.6°F (febrile)
• Pulse oximetry (if not already checked)	SpO_2 = 96% on room air/ 100% on O_2
• Glucose level	BG = 88 mg/dL
• Providers ask pertinent questions of patient.	Information obtained should include the SAMPLE history: • Signs and Symptoms: Persistent coughing • Allergies: None • Medications: Does not take any because she thinks the doctor is a quack • Past medical history: Doesn't like to go to the doctor • Last intake: Coffee for breakfast 2 hours ago • Events leading up: Coughing has become worse today

Section 4: Skill Stations

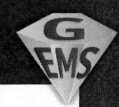

- Providers apply cardiac monitor.   Cardiac monitor shows normal sinus rhythm.
- Providers perform 12-lead ECG.   ECG shows normal sinus rhythm.

Management Strategies

What are your initial treatment priorities?

BLS priorities:
- Provide O_2.
- Carefully interview the patient to search for causes of the respiratory complaint (productive cough).
- Maintain a high index of suspicion for self-neglect or abuse.
- Move the patient to a warmer environment.

ALS priorities:
- BLS priorities plus:
  - Start an IV.
  - Maintain a high index of suspicion for self-neglect, hypothermia, hypoglycemia, and hypoxia.

If hypoglycemia is diagnosed by ALS crew:
- Administer dextrose (D_{50}), thiamine (depending on local protocol).
- Consider transport to an emergency department.
- 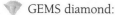 GEMS diamond:
  - G: Patient has persistent, productive cough that has lasted two weeks.
  - E: Newspapers and mail are stacked against the front door. Indoor environment is cold—38°F; heat appears to be off. Residence is filthy.
  - M: None
  - S: Patient lives at home alone. Patient is depressed over death of spouse, doesn't care about anything.

Issues in Management

Since one-third of the self-neglect patients have persistently refused offers of any help, an ethical dilemma confronts the EMS provider: whether or not to force treatment and care. This dilemma is compounded if there is a risk to the patients themselves, their families, the institution, or the community. This includes risks from fire, blocked sewers, accumulated rubbish, or a health threat. Although compulsory powers are rarely used, in some cases they are necessary, especially for those persons who develop severe physical problems (eg, pneumonia, stroke, heart failure, ulcers) or disabilities. In such cases, it may be justifiable to encourage, or possibly even force, admission to a hospital or nursing home. Local protocol should dictate the best care for the patient. In some states the police may have to get involved to put the patient under protective custody for the benefit of the patient's well being.

Also, it is important to remember to protect the patient's privacy. If the patient is wearing many layers of clothes and you need to expose him or her for the examination, expose only a small area at a time. Keep the patient's clothes or blankets on him or her to minimize heat loss.

Case Development

The patient has a productive cough with yellow phlegm and states that she (he) hasn't been eating regularly. The patient called you because the cough and fever have gotten worse over the past two days.

Core Knowledge Points

At the end of the call, tell the EMS team to provide a brief "radio style" report on the patient. After this is complete, ask the two observers to each give a report on what they observed during the call, and to specifically address the questions that they were asked to fill out on their form.

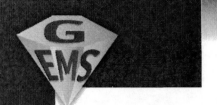

Section 4: Skill Stations

In this simulation, it is important to recognize the patient's unsuitable living conditions. Did the providers investigate why there was uncollected mail and newspapers? Did the providers ask why the patient neglected to seek medical attention earlier? These are signs of self- neglect. Point this out in class. Did the providers talk to the patient enough to get the patient to say that she (or he) was depressed, or did they stop asking before the patient felt comfortable enough to give that information? Give pointers for how the providers can communicate more effectively with the older patient who is depressed. This discussion should provide them with memorable, real, practical advice that they can use in the field.

What is good technique for interviewing an older patient?
- Direct questioning of the patient is the primary choice.
- Correlating and background information should be collected and later reported to the emergency department staff and social services.
- Correct positioning in the patient's line of sight and adequate voice tone are important.
- Allow adequate time for answers to questions.
- Avoid multiple questioners.

Summary

Self-neglect in the older population should be distinguished from neglect related to abuse or mistreatment. Neglect is caused by other people, but self-neglect is self-imposed, and in some cases a particular lifestyle is involved. Other names used for self-neglect in older people are Diogenes syndrome (DS), aged reclusion, social breakdown of the elderly, and squalor syndrome. DS is not related to mental disorders. It involves occurrences preceding a disease state, for example, precipitating factors such as the death of a spouse or a change in daily life, such as moving. Day care and community care are the main methods of management.[1]

When assessing the patient, the EMS provider should initially concentrate on other subjects of conversation, including the patient's history and background, rather than making an initial assault on the problem of self-neglect. The plan of care involves a balance between support and direct intervention. Other strategies are to increase family and social support. The management of this patient should primarily be assessment and treatment of the clinical presentation of possible pneumonia or respiratory complaint.

---

[1] *Annals of Long-Term Care: Clinical Care and Aging.* 2001;9[2]:21–24.

Section 4: Skill Stations

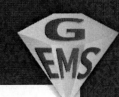

Skill Station #2: Immobilization

This 30-minute skill station will allow the students to practice immobilization of the older trauma patient, particularly using alternative methods for padding such as blankets, pillows, and other available devices, such as a vacuum mattress or commercial inflatable pillow. Two emergency situations are provided; you will use each of these situations.

Objectives

At the end of this station, the student will be able to:
- Assess each scenario in a systematic, consistent way.
- Explain the importance of proper communication with the older patient.
- Discuss the importance of maintaining a high index of suspicion for older trauma patients.
- Perform a comprehensive trauma exam to determine the presence of injuries.
- Utilize appropriate immobilization technique to minimize the negative effects of immobilization in the older patient.

Format

Student-Faculty ratio: six students per one Faculty member.

For each of the immobilization scenarios, one student will serve as the coached patient-actor. Three students will serve as the responding EMS crew. The remaining students will be observers and assist with the post-assessment critique led by the instructor.

Logistics

Station: 30 minutes
Breakdown:

2 min.	Faculty introduces format and expectations.
2 min.	**Situation #1:** 1st patient-actor taken aside, coached.
8 min.	Rescue crew assesses/packages patient.
5 min.	Assessment debriefing, review of key teaching points
2 min.	**Situation #2:** 2nd patient-actor chosen, taken aside, coached.
8 min.	2nd rescue crew assesses/packages patient.
5 min.	Debriefing, critique
2 min.	Wrap-up

Room Requirements

The room should be large enough to hold six students, the Faculty, and all the carry-in EMS equipment. The room should be quiet enough to permit interviewing and listening. There should be enough chairs and tables to accommodate the observing students. There should be enough space for the simulated patient to lay supine and be treated by the providers.

Equipment Needs

Notecards for simulation (provided in the GEMS Teaching Package and in this section)
Exam gloves (1 box each of large, medium, and small) (latex-free if possible)
Oxygen tank and oxygen administration supplies
First aid kit including blood pressure cuff, stethoscope
Long board
Scoop stretcher
Cervical collars
Head blocks/head bed immobilization device

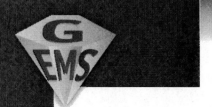

Section 4: Skill Stations

Straps/tape
Padding to fill void spaces (blankets, pillows, or commercial device)
Towels or small pillows (to simulate osteoporosis/kyphosis)
T-shirt
Medication bottles with simulated labels (Lasix, Lanoxin)
Stuffed animal cats/dogs
Sets of fake eggs and milk (can be drawn on a piece of paper, purchased in a toy store, or empty egg cartons and empty milk cartons)
Mouth guards or large gumballs (Note: For the course, you will need one mouth guard or gumball per student in total. If you opt to use the Additional Activities found on page 190, you will need additional mouth guards/gumballs.)
Earplugs (Note: For the course, you will need one pair of earplugs per student in total. If you opt to use the Additional Activities found on page 190, you will need additional pairs of earplugs.)
Patient simulation materials:
- Sunglasses with tape on lenses (can be plastic, nonprescription)
- Yellow-tinted (or other color) sunglasses

Or

- Geriatric simulation kit

Teaching Points

The Faculty will cover the following points during this skill station. Standard EMS assessment technique should be followed; however, the following should be considered in assessing the older patient:
- Communication technique is also important with the trauma patient.
- Hearing and speech impairment must be considered in older patients.
- Fall injury is the leading cause of traumatic death for older persons.
- Falls may occur as result of a cardiac event or medical condition.
- Older patients are at greater risk for major injury from trauma.
- Medications may mask normal signs of hypovolemic shock.
- Patients with history of hypertension may be in shock at "normal" blood pressures.
- Past medical history taking is important to discover co-morbidity factors.
- Older patients are at greater risk of injury from standard immobilization practices.
- Padding of voids due to kyphosis or other conditions will be necessary.
- Protection from hypothermia is important in the older trauma patient.

Section 4: Skill Stations

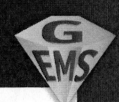

Situation #1

In Situation #1, one student simulates the patient, three students simulate the EMS team, and two students serve as observers.

On the following page, directions for each of the simulated parties are provided. These directions are provided as perforated cards in the GEMS Teaching Package for convenience. If you do not have the GEMS Teaching Package, before you teach the course, photocopy the instructions for each situation and cut them at the dotted lines. Distribute these to the students. Be sure to make enough photocopies for two skill sessions.

Give the glasses and earplugs to the student simulating the patient. Have the student put on the T-shirt. Place the towel or small pillow inside the back of the shirt, below the neck, to simulate kyphosis. Inform the student playing the patient to keep his or her head and shoulders flexed forward if possible to suggest kyphosis.

Once the student playing the simulated patient has had a chance to read his or her instruction card and has his or her props, have him or her lay on the floor. Place fake eggs, fake milk, and fake cats/dogs on the ground at the patient's feet.

Hand the dispatch information to one of the observing students to read out loud when you are ready to begin.

Tell the students to begin. Announce that they have 8 minutes to complete the call.

Half way through the call, announce that they are half way. Make a subsequent announcement when there are 2 minutes left.

Section 4: Skill Stations

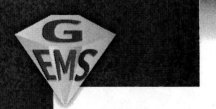

IMMOBILIZATION
Situation 1

Simulated Patient:
You will be a 78-year-old woman (or man) who lives at home alone. You are normally alert and able to care for yourself. You fell while in the kitchen making breakfast. *IF* providers ask about why you fell, you can't remember. Your chief complaint is pain in the right hip area. You should try to simulate right leg shortening/rotation. You should complain loudly of tenderness when moved, jostled, or even palpated in this area. Your past medical history is vague but includes a heart condition for which you take furosemide (Lasix) and digoxin (Lanoxin). Occasionally during assessment, you should voice reluctance to being transported, saying that if EMS could only help you into bed, you'd be okay. *IF* providers ask about why you're reluctant, you should say you're worried about your cats. Providers should help find an acceptable solution to this problem.

Props: The Faculty will provide you with glasses to simulate vision problems, earplugs to simulate hearing problems, and a T-shirt and towel or small pillow to simulate kyphosis.

IMMOBILIZATION
Situation 1

EMS Team:
You will be asked to assess and treat a simulated patient. As much as possible, obtain your information from the patient. Use a hands-on approach to this training exercise. Certain assessment information will be provided to you as your assessment progresses. For example, if you apply a BP cuff and simulate its inflation, you will be provided with the simulated blood pressure. You are to treat and package your patient to the point where the patient would be placed onto the gurney. At this point you will be asked to provide a brief "radio style" report on your patient.

IMMOBILIZATION
Situation 1

Dispatch Information:
You are a BLS (ALS) ambulance responding to a 78-year-old woman (man) who has fallen. You arrive to a modest but clean home in an older neighborhood. The patient lives alone and is unable to get up to the door. You are told the location of the "hidden key" and make access to the interior. The scene appears safe and you find your patient on the floor of a kitchen. There is spilled milk and eggs on the counter and floor and two cats (or dogs) are lapping at this mess.

Section 4: Skill Stations

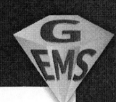

IMMOBILIZATION
Situation 1

Observing Students:
Your role in this situation is to observe the providers responding to the simulated call. Throughout the call, pay particular attention to what the providers did or did not do to address the patient's needs. As you are observing the call, fill out the following questions:

1. Did the providers try to speak with the patient?   _____ Yes   _____ No

_____

_____

2. Did the providers address the cats and spilled eggs and milk? If so, what did they do? If not, what could they have done?

_____

_____

3. Did they obtain a thorough history to determine when the patient fell?

_____

_____

4. What did they do differently to address the patient's kyphosis when backboarding the patient? Were they gentle in handling the patient?

_____

_____

5. What did they do to address the patient's emotional needs?

_____

_____

When the situation is finished, report your observances to the group.

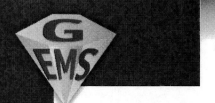

Section 4: Skill Stations

Initial Assessment/Focused History and Physical Exam

In this chart, information regarding the patient is provided in regular font. This information should be given to the students simulating the EMS crew if they ask for it. Possible interventions are provided in italics.

Assessment	Actions, Findings, and *Possible Interventions*
Scene Safety • The scene appears safe. • Providers take BSI precautions.	*Providers should verbalize caution about entry into a locked residence. Providers should deal with the cats (or dogs). Existence of mess on the floor may be seen as a safety hazard for EMS providers.*
Initial Assessment • Providers introduce selves and determine chief complaint.	*Providers properly position themselves at patient's level for direct communication.* Initial impression of patient: conscious, alert, and in discomfort.
• Airway	Airway is open.
• Breathing	Breathing is regular, non-labored.
• Circulation	Pulse is strong, slightly elevated.
• Mental status	Patient answers questions appropriately.

Focused History & Physical Exam
• Providers check vital signs:
  • Blood pressure
  • Pulse
  • Respirations
  • Lung sounds
  • Temperature
  • Pulse oximetry (if not already checked)
  • Glucose level
	
	BP = 156/102 mm Hg
	HR = 110 beats/min
	RR = 16 breaths/min
	Lung sounds = clear
	Temp = 97.2°F
	SpO_2 = 98% on room air
	BG = 92 mg/dL

• Providers ask pertinent questions of patient.	Information obtained should include the SAMPLE history: • Signs and Symptoms: Pain in right hip • Allergies: None • Medications: Lasix, Lanoxin • Past medical history: Unknown heart problem • Last intake: Patient was making breakfast when she fell. • Events leading up: Unknown
• Providers perform physical exam.	Brief exam starting from head shows no signs of injury until right pelvic/hip area is reached. Patient has tenderness to right hip area. Right leg is shortened and internally rotated. Distal pulse, motor, sensory are intact.
• Providers should apply cardiac monitor.	Cardiac monitor shows sinus tachycardia.

Section 4: Skill Stations

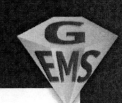

Management Strategies

What are your initial treatment priorities?

BLS priorities:
- Stabilize patient's situation to prevent further injury.
- Carefully interview the patient and caregiver (if available) to learn chief complaint and how fall occurred.
- Maintain a high index of suspicion for other injury or medical condition besides the chief complaint.
- Extricate/package patient to minimize movement and maximize comfort.
- Place a blanket on the board prior to immobilization.
- Utilize padding, tape, and straps to properly immobilize in a position of comfort.

ALS priorities:
- BLS priorities plus:
  - Consider the need for cardiac monitoring.
  - Consider the need for IV analgesia prior to patient immobilization.
  - Extricate/package patient to minimize movement and maximize comfort.
  - Place a blanket on the board prior to immobilization.
  - Utilize padding, tape, and straps to properly immobilize in a position of comfort.
- GEMS diamond:
  - G: Patient fell while making breakfast.
  - E: Home is modest but clean. There are spilled eggs and milk on the floor.
  - M: Patient takes Lasix and Lanoxin for a heart condition.
  - S: Patient lives at home alone. Patient is reluctant to be transported.

Issues in Management

This case represents a typically challenging EMS response to an older fall patient. As with incidents that are purely medical (as opposed to trauma), quality communication with older patients may require patience and good technique.

This case tries to get providers to think about why a fall has occurred and to search for an underlying medical explanation. The patient may have slipped or tripped or may have had a cardiac event which led to syncope and a fall. Medical history and medications may help explain why a fall occurred or may complicate the assessment and treatment. Falls in the older population are serious and EMS providers should not minimize their importance. Cardiac monitoring may reveal a previously unknown problem. Careful review of medication in the patient's home may uncover inappropriate medication usage.

Case Development

The EMS providers package the patient using a long board or scoop stretcher, along with padding and straps. Gentle technique must be used, as the skin and bones of an older patient are much frailer than those of a younger patient.

As they prepare for transport, they can verbalize that they would provide a brief clean up of the spilled mess. Also, they should obtain the patient's direction on how to care for the cats (or dogs) and ensure that this is addressed.

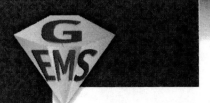

Section 4: Skill Stations

Core Knowledge Points

At the end of the call, tell the EMS team to provide a brief "radio style" report on the patient.
- Fall injury is a serious and common problem for older people.
- Falls may be caused by a medical event such as cardiac arrhythmia.
- Older patients are at higher risk for major injury from relatively minor trauma mechanisms.
- Medical history or medications may mask symptoms of injury.
- Immobilization of patients with hip fractures requires flexibility, patience, padding, and gentle technique.

Summary

Trauma in the older patient can have many causes ranging from an environmental problem such as a stair that is hard for the patient to see, to medication interactions, to a medical condition. It is extremely important to get as much information as possible to help determine the cause of the fall, as this may be related to the treatment and future prevention.

Remember that older patients have frailer skin and bones. Standard technique used by EMS providers may not be gentle enough for the older patient, and could result in discomfort or further injury to the patient. Technique must be adjusted to be as gentle as possible.

Backboards should be covered with a blanket or commercial pillow to minimize the discomfort at pressure points on an older patient's body. This padding will help spread pressure across the surface area and, combined with proper padding of the voids, will decrease the likelihood of pressure ulcers. Alternative immobilization devices, such as a vacuum mattress, may be used if allowed by local protocol.

Lastly, remember to address the social and emotional needs of the patient, such as ensuring that the patient's pets are cared for in his or her absence. These concerns are extremely important to patients, and addressing them are part of total patient care. Addressing them will also help the call run more smoothly, which is in everyone's best interest.

Section 4: Skill Stations

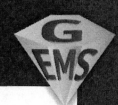

Situation #2

In Situation #2, one student simulates the patient, three students simulate the EMS team, and two students serve as observers.

On the following page, directions for each of the simulated parties are provided. These directions are provided as perforated cards in the GEMS Teaching Package for convenience. If you do not have the GEMS Teaching Package, before you teach the course, photocopy the instructions for each situation and cut them at the dotted lines. Distribute these to the students. Be sure to make enough photocopies for two skill sessions.

Give the earplugs and the mouth guard to the student simulating the patient. Have the student put on the T-shirt. Place the towel or small pillow inside the back of the shirt, below the neck, to simulate kyphosis. Inform the student playing the patient to keep his or her head and shoulders flexed forward if possible to suggest kyphosis.

Hand the dispatch information to one of the observing students to read out loud when you are ready to begin.

Tell the students to begin. Announce that they have 8 minutes to complete the call.

Half way through the call, announce that they are half way. Make a subsequent announcement when there are 2 minutes left.

Section 4: Skill Stations

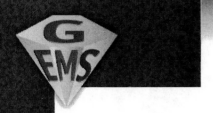

IMMOBILIZATION
Situation 2

Simulated Patient:
You will be an 85-year-old man (or woman) who was the driver in a vehicle that was hit head-on by a pickup truck. You are found lying on the sidewalk with your eyes closed. You cannot recall what happened and are somewhat dazed. You can provide your name and your address but can't recall the date and you're not sure where you are. You are not sure what hurts, but *IF* palpated, you have neck tenderness and chest tenderness. You deny shortness of breath. *IF* asked about medical history or medications, you should say you take a "heart blocker" and "a water pill."

Props: The Faculty will provide you with earplugs to simulate hearing problems, a mouth guard or gumball to simulate speech impairment, and a T-shirt and towel or small pillow to simulate kyphosis.

IMMOBILIZATION
Situation 2

EMS Team:
You will be asked to assess and treat a simulated patient. As much as possible, obtain your information from the patient. Use a hands-on approach to this training exercise. Certain assessment information will be provided to you as your assessment progresses. For example, if you apply a BP cuff and simulate its inflation, you will be provided with the simulated blood pressure. You are to treat and package your patient to the point where the patient would be placed onto the gurney. At this point, you will be asked to provide a brief "radio style" report on your patient.

IMMOBILIZATION
Situation 2

Dispatch and Arrival Information:
You are a BLS (ALS) ambulance responding to a motor vehicle collision. You arrive to a residential street where a pickup has struck a small car head on. The driver of the pickup denies injury. Your only patient is an older man (woman) lying on the sidewalk. You are told that someone helped him/her from the car. You note that his (her) car has a cracked windshield in front of the bent steering wheel. Damage to his (her) car is minor to moderate. The car did not have an airbag.

As you approach your patient you note that his (her) eyes are closed. You can see him (her) breathing, and you note an abrasion/hematoma to the forehead. The scene is safe.

Section 4: Skill Stations

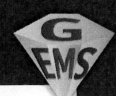

IMMOBILIZATION
Situation 2

Observing Students:

Your role in this situation is to observe the providers responding to the simulated call. Throughout the call, pay particular attention to what the providers did or did not do to address the patient's needs. As you are observing the call, fill out the following questions:

1. Did the providers try to speak with the patient? _____ Yes _____ No

_____
_____

2. Did they address life threats, if there were any?

_____
_____

3. Did they obtain a thorough history to determine when and how the patient crashed?

_____
_____

4. What did they do differently to address the patient's kyphosis when backboarding the patient? Were they gentle in handling the patient?

_____
_____

5. What did they do to address the patient's emotional needs?

_____
_____

When the situation is finished, report your observances to the group.

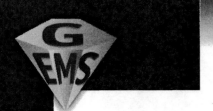

Section 4: Skill Stations

Initial Assessment/Focused History and Physical Exam

In this chart, information regarding the patient is provided in regular font. This information should be given to the students simulating the EMS crew if they ask for it. Possible interventions are provided in italics.

Assessment	Actions, Findings, and *Possible Interventions*
Scene Safety • The scene appears safe. • Providers take BSI precautions.	*Providers may verbalize caution about MVC scene safety in general.*
Initial Assessment • Providers introduce selves and determine the following:	*Providers properly position themselves at patient's level for direct communication.* Patient opens eyes to verbal contact.
• Airway	Airway is open.
• Breathing	Breathing is regular, slightly elevated.
• Circulation	Pulse is strong, slightly elevated.
• Mental status	Patient answers questions but appears "dazed." Patient is oriented to name and date but cannot recall what happened or where he/she is. Patient cannot offer chief complaint, is vague and confused.
Focused History & Physical Exam • Providers should ask about specific possible injuries.	If asked about neck pain, the patient should say that it is sore. Patient denies shortness of breath or other injury.

• Providers check vital signs:
  • Blood pressure
  • Pulse
  • Respirations
  • Lung sounds
  • Temperature
  • Pulse oximetry (if not already checked)
  • Glucose level
	BP = 100/72 mm Hg
	HR = 72 beats/min
	RR = 16 breaths/min
	Lung sounds = clear
	Temp = 97.2°F
	SpO_2 = 92% on room air
	BG = 92 mg/dL if checked

• Providers ask pertinent questions of patient.	Information obtained should include the SAMPLE history: • Signs and Symptoms: Neck and chest tenderness after physical exam • Allergies: None • Medications: Unknown "heart blocker" and "water pill" • Past medical history: Unknown why he takes the medications • Last intake: Unknown • Events leading up: He cannot remember where he was or what he was doing.

Section 4: Skill Stations

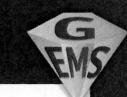

Assessment	Actions, Findings, and *Possible Interventions*
Focus History & Physical Exam (continued)	
• Providers perform physical exam.	**Physical Exam:** **Head:** Abrasion/hematoma on forehead. **Eyes:** PERL, no Battle's sign. **Face:** No facial deformity. Dentures intact and in place. **Neck:** Trachea midline, tenderness to palpation at about C4/5 level. **Chest:** Clavicles nontender. Patient has tenderness over sternum and some ribs. Breath sounds clear. **Abdomen:** Patient has tenderness in right upper quadrant. No rigidity. **Extremities:** Unremarkable. **Back:** Unremarkable. **Neuro:** Patient has pulse/motor/sensory intact ×4.
• Providers should apply cardiac monitor.	Cardiac monitor shows normal sinus rhythm with multiform premature ventricular contractions (PVCs) between 10–12/min.

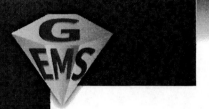
Section 4: Skill Stations

Management Strategies

What are your initial treatment priorities?

BLS priorities:
- Assess patient for life-threatening injuries.
- Protect and immobilize the patient's cervical spine.
- Administer supplemental oxygen.
- Determine the chief complaint and/or obvious injury.
- Maintain a high index of suspicion for major injury or medical condition besides the chief complaint.
- Decide whether the patient meets trauma system criteria for expedited treatment/transport.
- Package the patient to minimize movement and maximize comfort.
- Place a blanket on the board prior to immobilization.
- Utilize padding, tape, and straps to properly immobilize the patient in a position of comfort.
- Communicate with trauma system.

ALS priorities:
- BLS priorities plus:
  - Initiate IV(s) en route.

 GEMS diamond:
- G: Patient was hit head-on by a pick-up truck.
- E: The patient's windshield is cracked in front of the bent steering wheel. The patient's car did not have an airbag.
- M: Patient takes a heart blocker and a water pill.
- S: Nothing noted.

Issues in Management

This case represents a potentially seriously injured older patient. The response to trauma in older patients may be different than for younger patients due to the effects of aging and/or medication.

This case tries to encourage providers to maintain a high index of suspicion for injury regardless of the vital signs. In this case, the patient is at greater risk of intracranial head injury. The spine of an older patient is more likely to be injured due to osteoporosis and decreased flexibility. The patient is also more susceptible to chest and abdominal injury as well. The presence of medications such as beta blockers may prevent the normal reaction of tachycardia even if the patient is bleeding internally.

Case Development

The EMS providers package the patient using a long board or scoop stretcher, along with padding and straps. The providers should verbalize their understanding that this patient may have serious internal injury. Immobilization should therefore be expedited but padding should be used to fill voids between the patient's body and the immobilization device. When padding the voids of a patient with kyphotic curvature of the spine, extra care should be taken. Gentle technique must always be used, as older patients' skin and bones are much frailer than those of a younger patient.

Section 4: Skill Stations

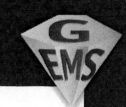

Core Knowledge Points

At the end of the call, tell the EMS team to provide a brief "radio style" report on the patient.

This patient's forehead hit the windshield and the patient's chest/abdomen hit the steering wheel. This should have been determined during the call, but if not, the instructor can tell this to the students now.

- Older patients are at higher risk for major injury from relatively minor trauma mechanisms.
- Medical history or medications may mask symptoms of injury.
- Spinal immobilization of patients requires flexibility, patience, padding, and gentle technique.
- Spinal immobilization may be aided with the use of commercial devices.

Summary

Spinal immobilization is an important skill to be mastered by all EMS providers. In the older patient, anatomical differences can necessitate the use of special techniques to appropriately immobilize the head, neck, and spine. Also, using a gentle technique is extremely important, so the older patient is not further injured or made uncomfortable during immobilization and transport.

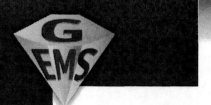

Section 4: Skill Stations

Optional ALS Skill Station: Intravenous Therapy

In this optional 60-minute skill station, each student will have the opportunity to observe the IV insertion procedure done correctly, handling the equipment and performing each skill while supervised. Procedure practice skills include:
- IV insertion
- Securing the IV

Intravenous (IV) therapy is an invasive procedure utilized to obtain venous access to the circulatory system. The most common method of gaining access is via the peripheral veins. Peripheral IV therapy involves the percutaneous insertion of an IV catheter into a peripheral vein.

In the older patient, this procedure is established for the following indications:
- To administer fluids for volume replacement
- To administer medications by either a bolus or to administer a drip
- To establish a lifeline for medication administration or volume replacement in case the patient's condition deteriorates

In the older patient, establishing vascular access is often difficult. There are physiological changes that must be recognized in attempting to initiate IV therapy. For example, there is no change in the epidermis in older people; however, the dermis undergoes major changes as a result of the aging process. This accounts for the laxity of the skin.

Inserting the IV catheter and puncturing the epidermis can cause a large hematoma. Smaller catheters such as 20-, 22-, or 24-gauge are preferable unless rapid fluid replacement is necessary. In the older patient, some commonly used medications have a tendency to create fragile skin. Before initiating the insertion of the catheter, it is important to ask the patient where access has been successfully started before. In the older patient who may have multiple chronic illnesses, their previous experiences can assist you in making a successful attempt.

Objectives

At the end of this station, the student will be able to:
- Demonstrate the technique used to insert an IV catheter on a simulated older patient.
- Identify different types of veins to avoid and veins on which to attempt IV access in the older patient.
- Recognize the need to secure the IV site completely but with care of the older patient's fragile skin.

Format

Student-Faculty ratio: six students per one Faculty member.

Logistics

Station: 60 minutes
Breakdown:

5 min.	Lead Faculty introduces the station to the students and states the skill objectives.
10 min.	Faculty demonstrates vascular access (IV skills).
30 min.	Each student performs IV therapy skills: • IV insertion • Securing the IV
15 min.	Faculty discusses Situation 1 and answers questions regarding skill and Situation 1.

Section 4: Skill Stations

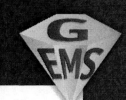

Room Requirements

The room should be large enough to hold six students, the Faculty, and all the carry-in EMS equipment including the IV insertion arms/hands. The room should be well lit. There should be several long tables on which to set up the IV insertion arms/hands. There should be seven chairs.

Equipment Needs

Exam gloves (1 box each) large, medium, and small. Latex-free if possible.
IV insertion arms or IV insertion hands
Towels or chucks to protect tables from spills
Goggles or protective eyewear
IV over-the-needle catheters (2 per student) (various sizes)
Tape for securing IV catheter
Scotch tape to fasten paper to dummy arm
Sharps containers with covers
Scissors to cut tape
Alcohol wipes and Betadine solution (cleansing agent)
Rubbing alcohol
4" × 4" non-sterile gauze (4 boxes)
IV fluid containers
IV administration sets (minidrip or macrodrip)
Venous constriction bands
Tissue paper to utilize as covering IV insertion tools to mimic fragile skin
Blood pressure cuff
2- or 4-inch Kling bandaging

Teaching Points

The Faculty will cover the following points during this skill station:
- Communication with the patient as the procedure is being performed, to make the older patient comfortable
- Skin concerns in the older patient, including the increased risk of bruising and the care needed to avoid skin tears
- Decreased ability of wounds to heal in the older patient. Utilize sterile techniques and cautious fluid administration at all times.
- Preparing equipment and having forethought will help in the prevention of errors while attempting IV therapy
- Assessment of the older patient for IV therapy indications and contraindications
- Assessment for correct placement, identification of complications after IV therapy is established, and changes in the patient's condition
- Accurate documentation of procedures performed
- Taking past medical history assessment to ascertain allergies or untoward effects of previous IV therapy attempts
- Communication of IV therapy procedures performed in the prehospital setting to the receiving emergency department personnel

Before conducting this skill station, prepare the IV insertion arms/hands by fastening tissue paper to them to simulate fragile older skin. The tissue paper can be covered with Vaseline and/or water to make it more fragile.

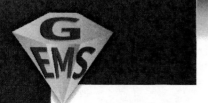

Section 4: Skill Stations

Skill Practice

Demonstrate proper IV therapy technique on one of the IV insertion arms/hands, reminding students of the special considerations in older patients. Students should do the following when performing IV therapy:
- Identify the signs and symptoms of dehydration.
- Try using smaller catheters (20-, 22-, or 24-gauge)
- Initiate IV insertion starting at hand, avoiding small spidery veins and varicose veins. Utilize sterile technique.
- Secure IV carefully with tape. Remind student that tape can lead to skin damage.
- Alternatively secure the IV with Kling bandage.
- Accurately document IV insertion.
- Consider need for cardiac monitoring.
- Maintain high index of suspicion for other underlying medical conditions, for example, sepsis, malnutrition, electrolyte imbalance, neglect, and cardiogenic shock.
- Keep the patient comfortable.

Let the students practice IV therapy on an IV insertion arm/hand.

Section 4: Skill Stations

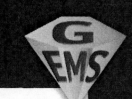

Situation #1

Read the following scenario once the students have practiced the IV therapy skill.
- You are dispatched to the apartment of 72-year-old woman who lives alone. The next door neighbor called, stating she hadn't seen her older neighbor in three days and was concerned.
- The manager of the apartment complex let you gain access to the patient. The scene is safe and providers take BSI precautions. You gain assess and find the patient in bed, stating, "I feel weak."

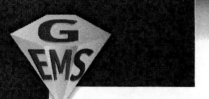

Section 4: Skill Stations

Initial Assessment/Focused History and Physical Exam

In this chart, information regarding the patient is provided in regular font. This information should be given to the students simulating the EMS crew if they ask for it. Possible interventions are provided in italics.

Assessment	Actions, Findings, and *Possible Interventions*
Scene Safety • The scene appears safe. • Providers take BSI precautions.	
Initial Assessment • Providers introduce selves and determine chief complaint.	*Providers properly position themselves at patient's level for direct communication.* Initial impression of patient: conscious, alert, weak
• Airway	Airway is open and patent.
• Breathing	Breathing is regular and unlabored.
• Circulation	Pulse is weak and thready.
• Mental status	Patient answers questions in full sentences and appropriately.

Focused History & Physical Exam
• Providers check vital signs:
  • Blood pressure
  • Pulse
  • Respirations
  • Lung sounds
  • Temperature
  • Pulse oximetry
  • Glucose level
	
	BP = 70/50 mm Hg
	HR = 110 beats/min
	RR = 18 breaths/min
	Lung sounds = clear bilaterally
	Temp = 99.6°F
	SpO2 = 98% on room air
	BG = 60 mg/dL

• Providers ask pertinent questions of patient.	Information obtained should include the SAMPLE history: • Signs and Symptoms: General weakness • Allergies: Medical tape • Medications: None • Past medical history: Diet-controlled diabetes • Last oral intake: Over 24 hours • Events leading up: Has been feeling sick for 3 days
• Providers perform physical exam.	No signs of trauma. Examination reveals (starting from the head) sunken eyes, dry mucosa, tenting of the skin, weak peripheral pulses, motor and sensory is intact.
• Providers should apply cardiac monitor.	Cardiac monitor shows sinus tachycardia without ectopy.

Section 4: Skill Stations

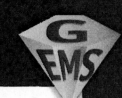

Management Strategies

What are your initial treatment priorities?

BLS priorities:
- Provide 100% oxygen (15 L/min) as tolerated.
- Accommodate patient's needs before transport, for example, obtain reading glasses, dentures, and personal items to take with the patient.
- Transport the patient in position of comfort and/or assist ALS providers.

ALS priorities:
- BLS priorities plus:
  - Monitor the patient for deterioration.
  - Attempt intravenous access.
  - Fluid resuscitation (200 mL bolus for this patient)
  - Initiate cardiac monitoring.

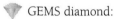 GEMS diamond:
- G: Patient is in bed, feels weak.
- E: Nothing noted.
- M: None.
- S: Patient lives at home alone. Neighbor hadn't seen patient in three days and was concerned. Manager of apartment complex appears helpful.

Issues in Management

In this situation, a through investigation of the chief complaint is vital. Good communication is paramount, and requires patience and good patient assessment technique.

This case enables the providers to focus on a detailed history and search for an underlying medical condition. Medical history-taking will reveal that this patient has diabetes. She has not had oral intake or nutriment, leading the providers to suspect dehydration or an electrolyte imbalance. As a patient advocate for older people, the providers cannot rule out neglect. Cardiac monitoring is essential to rule out any cardiac anomaly.

When discussing this scenario, remind students of the following important points when performing IV therapy:
- Assess the need for oxygen therapy.
- Avoid varicose veins and spidery veins.
- Check IV site for extravasation. If this occurs, immediately disconnect IV and apply cold compress to reduce swelling and hematoma.
- Conduct a complete focused exam and history taking.
- Document living conditions for social work referral and notification.
- Initiate fluid resuscitation.
- Check blood glucose levels.
- Carefully secure IV.
- Transport the patient in position of comfort.

Case Development

The patient responded positively to oxygen therapy and a 200 mL fluid resuscitation bolus. Her blood pressure increased to 90/60 mm Hg. She responds to 25 g of D_{50}. A patent IV was established to the right hand metacarpal vein (in the patient's own words, "It wasn't bad at all") with the insertion of a 20-gauge catheter. The IV site was secured using Kling bandaging in order to avoid an allergic reaction to the tape. The manager of the apartment complex is informed that the patient will be transported to the emergency department for further evaluation. He will secure the apartment and notify relatives.

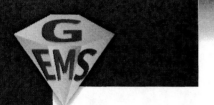

Section 4: Skill Stations

Core Knowledge Points

Older patients who are chronically ill may present with multiple complaints. Medical history and medication adherence may mask sign and symptoms.

One of the basic principles of infusion therapy in the older patient is to choose the smallest gauge catheter and place it in the largest vein. Blood can be infused through a 22-gauge catheter, although a larger IV is preferred for that purpose. Smaller catheters cause less damage to the vein wall and allow flow around the catheter. This leads to less phlebitis and longer dwell time.

Sterile technique should always be paramount in the older patient who may have a suppressed immune system.

Summary

- IV therapy is a skill that must be mastered by all prehospital care providers.
- BLS and ALS providers must be able to recognize the physiological changes that occur in older people, specifically the possible complications of IV therapy, such as local reactions (infiltration and phlebitis), or systemic complications including fluid overload or allergic reactions.
- Anatomical changes will necessitate slight adjustments in IV therapy procedures.

References

Andolsek, C.M. *Intravenous Therapy for Prehospital Providers*. Sudbury, MA: Jones and Bartlett, 2001.
Hadaway L, Gauging I.V. needle size. Nursing 2002, The Journal of Clinical Excellence, 2002. Volume 32, (7) 10–12.

Appendix

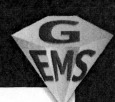

Section 5

Contents

GEMS BLS Course Fact Sheet..................................	232
GEMS ALS Course Fact Sheet..................................	233
Course Notification Form.....................................	234
Course Coordinator Application	235
Course Coordinator Orientation Session Confirmation Letter........	237
Faculty Confirmation Letter	238
Participant Confirmation Letter	239
GEMS Faculty Evaluation Form................................	241
GEMS Participant Evaluation Form.............................	243
GEMS Course Roster	245

Section 5: Appendix

GEMS BLS Course Fact Sheet

Course	Geriatric Education for Emergency Medical Services (GEMS) Basic Life Support (BLS) Course
Length	8 hours excluding breaks and lunch
Intended Audience	Professionals currently serving as Basic Life Support (BLS) providers (ie, First Responders and EMT-Basics)
Lectures	• Aging • Changes with Age • Communicating with Older People and Their Caregivers • Assessment of the Older Patient and Pharmacology • End-of-Life Care Issues • Trauma, Musculoskeletal Disorders, and Falls • Neurological Emergencies and Altered Mental Status • Respiratory and Cardiovascular Emergencies • Elder Abuse and Neglect
Scenarios	• Communication Challenges • Do Not Resuscitate Orders • Stroke • Medication Interactions • Dementia vs. Delirium • Elder Abuse and Neglect
Skills Practiced	• Conducting a Patient Assessment Interview • Immobilization
Materials	Each participant is required to have a copy of the GEMS Textbook.
Successful Completion	Participants who successfully complete the GEMS BLS course will receive a GEMS Course Completion Card, valid for two years. To successfully complete the course, the participant must: • Participate in the entire course • Successfully complete a 20-item, multiple-choice exam with a score of 80% (16 correct out of 20 questions)

GEMS ALS Course Fact Sheet

Course	Geriatric Education for Emergency Medical Services (GEMS) Advanced Life Support (ALS) Course
Length	9 hours and 30 minutes excluding breaks and lunch
Intended Audience	Professionals currently serving as Advanced Life Support (ALS) providers (ie, EMT-Intermediates, EMT-Paramedics, and higher), but other levels may be admitted at the Course Coordinator's discretion
Lectures	• Aging • Changes with Age • Communicating with Older People and Their Caregivers • Assessment of the Older Patient • End-of-Life Care Issues • Trauma, Musculoskeletal Disorders, and Falls • Neurological Emergencies and Altered Mental Status • Respiratory and Cardiovascular Emergencies • Elder Abuse and Neglect • Pharmacology and Medication Toxicity Emergencies • Psychiatric Emergencies
Scenarios	• Communication Challenges • Do Not Resuscitate Orders • Stroke • Medications Interactions • Dementia vs. Delirium • Elder Abuse and Neglect
Skills Practiced	• Conducting a Patient Assessment Interview • Immobilization
Materials	Each participant is required to have a copy of the GEMS Textbook.
Successful Completion	Participants who successfully complete the GEMS ALS course will receive a GEMS Course Completion Card, valid for two years. To successfully complete the course, the participant must: • Participate in the entire course • Successfully complete a 25-item, multiple-choice exam with a score of 80% (20 correct out of 25 questions)

Section 5: Appendix

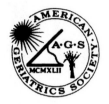 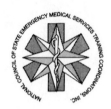

American Geriatrics Society
National Council of State EMS Training Coordinators
Geriatric Education for Emergency Medical Services (GEMS)
Course Notification Form

If you would like us to list this course on the GEMS website and refer individuals to your upcoming GEMS course, please complete this form by going to the GEMS website at www.GEMSsite.com. If you do not have internet access, please complete this form and mail or fax to:

GEMS
American Geriatrics Society
The Empire State Building
350 Fifth Avenue
Suite 801
New York, NY 10118
Fax: 212-832-8646

Course Coordinator: _____ **ID #:** _____

GEMS course being taught: ☐ BLS   ☐ ALS   ☐ Course Coordinator Orientation

Start date of course: _____

End date of course: _____

Location of course (include address, city, state, zip): _____
_____

Registration phone: _____

Registration E-mail: _____

Section 5: Appendix

American Geriatrics Society
National Council of State EMS Training Coordinators
Geriatric Education for Emergency Medical Services (GEMS)
Course Coordinator Application

Complete this form and submit it to the Course Coordinator who is conducting the Course Coordinator Orientation Session. If you are completing the Online Course Coordinator Orientation Session, this application can be submitted from the GEMS website at www.GEMSsite.com.

Applicant Information

(Please type or print clearly in dark ink.)

Name: _____
Medical Designation(s): _____
Title: _____
Institution/Employer: _____
Business Address: _____
City: _____ State: _____ Zip: _____
Home Address: _____
City: _____ State: _____ Zip: _____
Preferred Mailing Address (select one): ☐ Business ☐ Home
Work Phone: _____ Home Phone: _____
Other Phone: _____ Fax: _____
E-Mail (required): _____

GEMS Course Coordinator Requirements

Individuals who wish to be a GEMS Course Coordinator must meet the following requirements:
- Be a physician (MD or DO), registered nurse, nurse practitioner, advanced practice nurse, physician assistant, paramedic, or EMT with a background in EMS. Must be at least a paramedic to coordinate a GEMS ALS course.
- Successfully complete the GEMS provider course at the same or higher level for which the individual seeks to conduct courses.
- Submit the Course Coordinator application for approval to the Course Coordinator conducting the Course Coordinator Orientation Session or submit Course Coordinator application online at www.GEMSsite.com before completing the Online Course Coordinator Orientation Session.
- Have demonstrated experience in coordinating other nationally recognized standardized course for prehospital personnel. Have knowledge, experience, and expertise in the conduct of other adult education programs.
- Demonstrate an understanding and a working knowledge of the most recent GEMS course materials and policies.
- Complete a Course Coordinator Orientation Session from a GEMS Course Coordinator or the Online Course Coordinator Orientation Session at www.GEMSsite.com.

GEMS Course Coordinator Level

I am applying to become a GEMS Course Coordinator for the following GEMS courses:
(Reminder: Individuals must be at least a paramedic to coordinate a GEMS ALS course.)
☐ BLS
☐ ALS

Section 5: Appendix

Medical Education

I am a(n) (please **check all** that apply):
___ Physician. Describe your EMS involvement: _____
___ Registered Nurse. Describe your EMS involvement: _____
___ Nurse Practitioner. Describe your EMS involvement: _____
___ Physician Assistant. Describe your EMS involvement: _____
___ Emergency Medical Technician—Paramedic
___ Emergency Medical Technician—Intermediate
___ Emergency Medical Technician—Basic
___ Other (**must specify**): _____

Teaching Experience

Do you have experience coordinating another nationally recognized standardized course for teaching pre-hospital personnel? (select one)
☐ Yes   ☐ No

Please briefly describe your teaching experience below. Include other nationally recognized standardized courses that you have taught.
_____
_____
_____

GEMS Provider Course Completion Information

I successfully completed the GEMS provider course:
Please check one: ☐ BLS   ☐ ALS
Date of course:_____
Location of course:_____ City:_____ State:_____
Course Coordinator for Course:_____

NOTE:
Course Coordinator: If you were not the Faculty for the candidate's GEMS provider course, please verify the above information from the candidate's GEMS Course Completion Card. This form must accompany a completed GEMS roster, on which all Course Coordinator candidates are listed.

I verify that the information above is correct. I have read the information in the GEMS Resource Manual regarding the responsibilities of the GEMS Course Coordinator and am prepared to fulfill these responsibilities. I will maintain the integrity of the GEMS course by agreeing to ensure that the course is taught as presented in the GEMS materials.	I have reviewed this application and verify that the applicant meets the established requirements to be a GEMS Course Coordinator.
Applicant's Signature Date	Course Coordinator's Signature Date

An electronic version of this form can be located on the GEMS website at www.GEMSsite.com.

Section 5: Appendix

Course Coordinator Orientation Session Confirmation Letter

This is a sample Course Coordinator Orientation Session confirmation letter to be sent to individuals who are enrolled in a Course Coordinator Orientation Session. It is also available on the GEMS website at www.GEMSsite.com. The information in italics needs to be customized for your course.

Date

Name
Title
Institution
Address
City, State, Zip

Dear *name of GEMS provider:*

Thank you for enrolling in the GEMS Course Coordinator Orientation Session to be held at *name of location* in *city, state* on *date*.

The enclosed Course Coordinator application lists the requirements for becoming a GEMS Course Coordinator. Please come to the orientation with documentation of:

- Status as a physician, registered nurse, nurse practitioner, advanced practice nurse, physician assistant, paramedic, or EMT
- Successful completion of the GEMS provider course
- Experience coordinating other nationally recognized standardized courses for prehospital personnel

Please bring your GEMS Textbook to the orientation. *Enclose a GEMS Resource Manual or provide information on how they can obtain a GEMS Resource Manual.*

I look forward to meeting you at the GEMS Course Coordinator Orientation Session. Please contact me at *phone and/or e-mail* if you have questions about the orientation.

Sincerely,

Name of Course Coordinator
Title
Enclosures

Section 5: Appendix

Faculty Confirmation Letter

This is a sample Faculty confirmation letter to be sent to each Faculty member by the Course Coordinator. It is also available on the GEMS website at www.GEMSsite.com. The information in italics needs to be customized for your course.

Date

Name
Title
Institution
Address
City, State, Zip

Dear *name of Faculty member*:

Thank you for accepting the invitation to serve as a Faculty member for the Geriatric Education for Emergency Medical Services (GEMS) course that will be sponsored by *name of institution* and held in *city, state*.

You have agreed to teach the following portions of the GEMS course:
Topic
Date
Time
Location

A course schedule is enclosed for your reference. *Provide information on how the Faculty member can obtain a copy of the GEMS Textbook and Resource Manual or assure him/her that you will provide this in advance of the course. Provide information on when the Faculty member will have access to the slides for the appropriate lecture topic.*

Provide information about travel and lodging arrangements (if appropriate). Provide instructions on how to get to the course site, where to park, etc.

If you have questions about the content of your lecture topic or course logistics, please feel free to contact me at *phone number and/or e-mail address*. Thank you again for agreeing to participate in the upcoming GEMS course. I look forward to working with you at the course.

Sincerely,

Name of Course Coordinator
Title
Enclosures

Section 5: Appendix

Participant Confirmation Letter

This is a sample participant confirmation letter to be sent to each registrant for the GEMS course. It is also available on the GEMS website at www.GEMSsite.com. The information in italics needs to be customized for your course.

Date

Name
Title
Institution
Address
City, State, Zip

Dear *name of registrant:*

Thank you for registering for the Geriatric Education for Emergency Medical Services (GEMS) course, which will be held *dates* in *city, state*. This letter will provide information regarding course logistics, content, materials, and course preparation.

The course will be held at *name of location. Provide information on making travel and hotel arrangements if necessary. Provide directions to the course location and parking information. Instruct registrants where to check-in each day.*

A course schedule is enclosed. The course includes case-based lectures, scenarios, and skill stations. *Enclose a copy of the GEMS Textbook or provide the registrant with information on how to obtain a copy of the GEMS Textbook. Encourage registrant to review the GEMS Textbook prior to the course.*

To qualify to receive a GEMS Course Completion Card, you must participate in the entire GEMS course and successfully complete a written exam at the end of the course.

Provide any necessary information on course cancellation policies.

I look forward to meeting you at the GEMS course. If you have any questions about the course, you can contact me at *phone number and/or e-mail address.*

Sincerely,

Name of Course Coordinator
Title
Enclosures

Section 5: Appendix

American Geriatrics Society
National Council of State EMS Training Coordinators
Geriatric Education for Emergency Medical Services (GEMS)
Faculty Evaluation Form

Which GEMS course did you teach? ____ BLS ____ ALS

Please rate the content presented for each of the following sessions. Please circle your response.

Portion of Course	Not At All Useful	Fairly Useful	Very Useful	Extremely Useful	Not Used
Lecture: Aging	1	2	3	4	X
Video: Aging	1	2	3	4	X
Lecture: Changes with Age	1	2	3	4	X
Video: Communication and Assessment	1	2	3	4	X
Lecture: Communicating with Older People and Their Caregivers	1	2	3	4	X
BLS Lecture: Assessment of the Older Patient and Pharmacology	1	2	3	4	X
ALS Lecture: Assessment of the Older Patient	1	2	3	4	X
Scenario: Communication Challenges	1	2	3	4	X
Skill Station: Conducting a Patient Assessment Interview	1	2	3	4	X
Lecture: End-of-Life Care Issues	1	2	3	4	X
Lecture: Trauma, Musculoskeletal Disorders, and Falls	1	2	3	4	X
Video: Immobilization	1	2	3	4	X
Lecture: Neurological Emergencies and Altered Mental Status	1	2	3	4	X
Scenarios: Do Not Resuscitate Orders and Stroke	1	2	3	4	X
Skill Station: Immobilization	1	2	3	4	X
Lecture: Respiratory and Cardiovascular Emergencies	1	2	3	4	X
Lecture: Elder Abuse and Neglect	1	2	3	4	X
ALS Lecture: Pharmacology and Medication Toxicity Emergencies	1	2	3	4	X
ALS Lecture: Psychiatric Emergencies	1	2	3	4	X
Scenarios: Dementia vs. Delirium, Elder Abuse and Neglect, and Medication Interactions	1	2	3	4	X
ALS Video: Intravenous Therapy	1	2	3	4	X

Section 5: Appendix

Are there additional topics you would like to see added to the GEMS course?

Please provide your response to each of the following statements. Please circle your response.

Statement	Strongly Disagree	Disagree	Agree	Strongly Agree
The GEMS Resource Manual provided adequate information for conducting the lectures.	1	2	3	4
The GEMS Resource Manual provided adequate information for conducting the scenarios.	1	2	3	4
The GEMS Resource Manual provided adequate information for conducting the skill stations.	1	2	3	4
The GEMS Textbook provided adequate clinical information to teach the GEMS course.	1	2	3	4
The GEMS Textbook provided adequate practical information to properly care for geriatric patients.	1	2	3	4

Comments:

Section 5: Appendix

American Geriatrics Society
National Council of State EMS Training Coordinators
Geriatric Education for Emergency Medical Services (GEMS)
Participant Evaluation Form

Which GEMS course did you attend? _____ BLS _____ ALS

Please provide your feedback on how useful each portion of the course was to you. Please circle your response.

Portion of Course	Not At All Useful	Fairly Useful	Very Useful	Extremely Useful	Not Used
Lecture: Aging	1	2	3	4	X
Video: Aging	1	2	3	4	X
Lecture: Changes with Age	1	2	3	4	X
Video: Communication and Assessment	1	2	3	4	X
Lecture: Communicating with Older People and Their Caregivers	1	2	3	4	X
BLS Lecture: Assessment of the Older Patient and Pharmacology	1	2	3	4	X
ALS Lecture: Assessment of the Older Patient	1	2	3	4	X
Scenario: Communication Challenges	1	2	3	4	X
Skill Station: Conducting a Patient Assessment Interview	1	2	3	4	X
Lecture: End-of-Life Care Issues	1	2	3	4	X
Lecture: Trauma, Musculoskeletal Disorders, and Falls	1	2	3	4	X
Video: Immobilization	1	2	3	4	X
Lecture: Neurological Emergencies and Altered Mental Status	1	2	3	4	X
Scenarios: Do Not Resuscitate Orders and Stroke	1	2	3	4	X
Skill Station: Immobilization	1	2	3	4	X
Lecture: Respiratory and Cardiovascular Emergencies	1	2	3	4	X
Lecture: Elder Abuse and Neglect	1	2	3	4	X
ALS Lecture: Pharmacology and Medication Toxicity Emergencies	1	2	3	4	X
ALS Lecture: Psychiatric Emergencies	1	2	3	4	X
Scenarios: Dementia vs. Delirium, Elder Abuse and Neglect, and Medication Interactions	1	2	3	4	X
ALS Video: Intravenous Therapy	1	2	3	4	X

Section 5: Appendix

Please provide your response to each of the following statements.

Statement	Strongly Disagree	Disagree	Agree	Strongly Agree
This course taught me how to adjust my emergency management so that it is appropriate for the older patient.	1	2	3	4
I learned how to adjust my communication skills in order to maximize the information I receive, and attend to the patient's emotional as well as physical needs.	1	2	3	4
The GEMS Textbook was useful in preparation for the GEMS course.	1	2	3	4
The course inspired me to think of ways to improve the lives of older patients.	1	2	3	4
I feel differently towards older patients than before I took this course.	1	2	3	4
I plan to share the information or skills I learned with someone else.	1	2	3	4

Comments:

Section 5: Appendix

GEMS Course Roster

This form can be completed and submitted online for no charge by going to the GEMS web site at www.GEMSsite.com. There is a $20 processing fee for submitting the form via fax or mail.

Please enclose a check or provide a credit card number. Check # _____ Credit Card # _____ expiration date _____

(DO NOT WRITE IN THIS BOX)

| Rec'd | Entered: | Mailed: | C: | Course Date: |

GERIATRIC EDUCATION FOR EMERGENCY MEDICAL SERVICES (GEMS)
COURSE REPORT FORM

American Geriatrics Society

REMEMBER: TYPE OR PRINT CLEARLY IN DARK INK   **COMPLETE ALL FIELDS**

Course Information

Type of Course:	Please Check One	☐ BLS			☐ ALS				☐ Course Coordinator Orientation
Starting Date of Course:		MM	DD	YY	Ending Date of Course:		MM	DD	YY

Organization Sponsoring the Course: _____

Course Coordinator Information

Course Coordinator ID Number: _____

Name of Course Coordinator: _____

Address: _____

Phone: ( ) _____

E-mail: _____

Mail provider cards to above address. ☐ Other: _____

Course Coordinator's Signature: _____ Date _____

MAIL TO: American Geriatrics Society, GEMS Coordinator, The Empire State Building, 350 Fifth Avenue, Suite 801, New York, NY 10118

Section 5: Appendix

Faculty Information

Faculty's Name	Mailing Address	Phone	Credentials
			☐ MD ☐ EMT-P ☐ RN ☐ EMT-I ☐ PA ☐ EMT-B ☐ Other
			☐ MD ☐ EMT-P ☐ RN ☐ EMT-I ☐ PA ☐ EMT-B ☐ Other
			☐ MD ☐ EMT-P ☐ RN ☐ EMT-I ☐ PA ☐ EMT-B ☐ Other
			☐ MD ☐ EMT-P ☐ RN ☐ EMT-I ☐ PA ☐ EMT-B ☐ Other
			☐ MD ☐ EMT-P ☐ RN ☐ EMT-I ☐ PA ☐ EMT-B ☐ Other
			☐ MD ☐ EMT-P ☐ RN ☐ EMT-I ☐ PA ☐ EMT-B ☐ Other
			☐ MD ☐ EMT-P ☐ RN ☐ EMT-I ☐ PA ☐ EMT-B ☐ Other
			☐ MD ☐ EMT-P ☐ RN ☐ EMT-I ☐ PA ☐ EMT-B ☐ Other
			☐ MD ☐ EMT-P ☐ RN ☐ EMT-I ☐ PA ☐ EMT-B ☐ Other
			☐ MD ☐ EMT-P ☐ RN ☐ EMT-I ☐ PA ☐ EMT-B ☐ Other

Section 5: Appendix

	☐ MD ☐ RN ☐ PA ☐ Other	☐ EMT-P ☐ EMT-I ☐ EMT-B	☐ MD ☐ RN ☐ PA ☐ Other	☐ EMT-P ☐ EMT-I ☐ EMT-B	☐ MD ☐ RN ☐ PA ☐ Other	☐ EMT-P ☐ EMT-I ☐ EMT-B	☐ MD ☐ RN ☐ PA ☐ Other	☐ EMT-P ☐ EMT-I ☐ EMT-B	☐ MD ☐ RN ☐ PA ☐ Other	☐ EMT-P ☐ EMT-I ☐ EMT-B	☐ MD ☐ RN ☐ PA ☐ Other	☐ EMT-P ☐ EMT-I ☐ EMT-B

Section 5: Appendix

Participant Information

Participant's Name	Address	Phone	Pass	Fail	Credentials
			P	F	☐ EMT-B ☐ EMT-I ☐ EMT-P ☐ Other, please specify _____
			P	F	☐ EMT-B ☐ EMT-I ☐ EMT-P ☐ Other, please specify _____
			P	F	☐ EMT-B ☐ EMT-I ☐ EMT-P ☐ Other, please specify _____
			P	F	☐ EMT-B ☐ EMT-I ☐ EMT-P ☐ Other, please specify _____
			P	F	☐ EMT-B ☐ EMT-I ☐ EMT-P ☐ Other, please specify _____
			P	F	☐ EMT-B ☐ EMT-I ☐ EMT-P ☐ Other, please specify _____
			P	F	☐ EMT-B ☐ EMT-I ☐ EMT-P ☐ Other, please specify _____

Section 5: Appendix

	P	F	
			☐ EMT-B ☐ EMT-I ☐ EMT-P ☐ Other, please specify _____

	P	F	
			☐ EMT-B ☐ EMT-I ☐ EMT-P ☐ Other, please specify _____

	P	F	
			☐ EMT-B ☐ EMT-I ☐ EMT-P ☐ Other, please specify _____

	P	F	
			☐ EMT-B ☐ EMT-I ☐ EMT-P ☐ Other, please specify _____

	P	F	
			☐ EMT-B ☐ EMT-I ☐ EMT-P ☐ Other, please specify _____

	P	F	
			☐ EMT-B ☐ EMT-I ☐ EMT-P ☐ Other, please specify _____

	P	F	
			☐ EMT-B ☐ EMT-I ☐ EMT-P ☐ Other, please specify _____

Section 5: Appendix

	P	F	☐ EMT-B ☐ EMT-I ☐ EMT-P ☐ Other, please specify _____
	P	F	☐ EMT-B ☐ EMT-I ☐ EMT-P ☐ Other, please specify _____
	P	F	☐ EMT-B ☐ EMT-I ☐ EMT-P ☐ Other, please specify _____
	P	F	☐ EMT-B ☐ EMT-I ☐ EMT-P ☐ Other, please specify _____
	P	F	☐ EMT-B ☐ EMT-I ☐ EMT-P ☐ Other, please specify _____
	P	F	☐ EMT-B ☐ EMT-I ☐ EMT-P ☐ Other, please specify _____
	P	F	☐ EMT-B ☐ EMT-I ☐ EMT-P ☐ Other, please specify _____